Happy &

Gluten Free -

Lifestyle Guide

Fast Track to Happy Gluten Free
Life & Healing of Gluten Intolerance

Written By:

I0424106

Anne Peterson

Sifu William Lee

Author of several Amazon Bestsellers

Table of Contents

Foreword

There is hardly anything more annoying than long, draggy introduction to a book or movie. We'll going to make this one short, possibly sweet for most. *This isn't a cookbook;* it's a practical guide for living full, healthy and happy Gluten Free life. Recipes we all need and yet, one can get them everywhere. What you can't easily find are facts, tips, shortcuts, remedies and solutions – that is why we decided to write this book.

We are sure about potency of this work – it may assist you, teach and inspire you and most importantly, save your time and money by stopping you from running in to (quite) few mistakes.

If you are new to gluten free diet and lifestyle you will love it. If you are already adjusted to living without gluten you will be (most probably) surprised. In either case, these unique approaches to gluten free lifestyle and possible healing of the gluten intolerance, allergy to gluten or even celiac is rich with potency and practical value. Not only modern medicine considers healing celiac and gluten intolerance practically impossible, but also we can witness strong and profound endeavor to block and discredit attempts to promote possible remedies and/or ways out of gluten intolerance.

This book is not only providing relief but it's also explaining natural and easy way to diminish the symptoms and gradually heal from gluten intolerance. Sifu William Lee is known for his potent and easy to apply methods that make sound of Traditional Chinese Medicine stop being perceived as 'scary', foggy and complicated. This guide contains a video instructional that will make this clear as a sunny day.

Why Listen To Us?

We will give you very short and clear answer. We admit that this type of collaboration is not seen often, so it deserves a bit of explanation anyhow:

Before that, let us start by simple line; you can find a lot of gluten free recipes all around but this is not a recipe book. We see a great need for practical guide to painless and happy Gluten free lifestyle.

About Anne Peterson

"In answer to the above question, ("why listen to these authors...") there are quite few reasons you could find strong and valid. There is probably one reason that dominates all others. Few decades of Veganism and consulting experience are great but having two children, both suffering from two different forms of sensitivity to Gluten does make a difference. On top of that during mid 80's not many people (including the medical personal) knew much about hypersensitivity to Gluten and related conditions, right? Long story short, being affectionate and loving mother dedicated to understand the matter and find the best way to help their children makes Anne 'authority' in this field. Not a doctor, not a professor but a real and authentic expert.

I am very happy we have met on time. Accepting any client, especially young mother with two kinds, boy and the girl that suffer is a challenge. I am so pleased I have accepted that challenge and despite of the complexity I did not turned away from that chance. I have learned many things due to our relationship that grew over the years. One of the amazing discoveries I got to is how modern alternative approach is not at all distant from the views of Traditional Chinese Medicine if you just know how to compare them".

Written by Sifu William Lee, 2nd March 2015, Zhengzhou, China

About Sifu William Lee

"It is very difficult for me to fit answer on this question in just few lines. Sifu Lee is just personification of advanced science and practices related to TCM (Traditional Chinese Medicine) that aren't at all simple to understand and yet he is teaching everything in a way that is so easy to understand and apply. Everyone familiar with his books knows that and no one of his readers or students need any introduction. I have enormous amount of respect and gratefulness towards him and his work – without his help I would experience a lot longer way to solutions I had to find for my family. In this world, people like Sifu Lee are extremely rare gems.

Now, if you do not know much about him, let me share you one thing with you. His approach to anything, as well as to matters of healing and health is hitting the root cause of the problems. He is not wasting any time and energy with theoretical explanations and such but is dealing with the very cause of a problem – that is fantastic! And one more thing – you know that Chinese proverb "If you want to help to hungry man do not feed him but teach him to fish..." THAT exactly is what Sifu Lee is all about and I have no words to express my gratefulness for everything he did and for willing to co author this book with me."

Written by Anne Peterson, 4th March 2015, Fairfield, Iowa, US

Why This Book?

Using just few words, answer would be "in order to help you avoid mistakes and save (a lot of) your time, energy and MONEY!" You probably already have your own experience – things that are complicated, normally are not effective and are simply just too demanding. For person suffering from gluten intolerance, there is no limit of choices – there are so many diet plans, cook books, information ... that may sometimes be really confusing. Yes, fact is that man and women affected with celiac disease are not alone. Different support groups are active in giving support and there are other sides that offer the support yet it is very important to know *whom to listen and who better not – similarly there are those from whom advice we better stay away.*

In this book therefore, you can get all the information related to celiac disease, gluten intolerance and gluten allergy you need to know as well as the easiest ways of living with gluten sensitivity without pain and struggle. Unique element of this book is the part where remedy and potential healing of the gluten intolerance is explained. Because of the Sifu Lee's expert insight, ancient methods of Traditional Chinese Medicine are here to guarantee you the efficiency and simplicity.

You will also get comprehensive but easy to understand information about:

-Deeper insights in the celiac disease disorder, gluten intolerance and allergy to gluten
-Complications accompanying those that are affected with gluten intolerance
-Treatments and remedies
-Myths and (popular) false understandings in relation to gluten intolerance...

Now just few more words about unique thing are that you just can't find elsewhere. In our guide, you will find simple yet powerful routine, presented in Amazon bestselling books authored by Sifu William Lee. Book Total Chi Fitness is explaining these methods in details, yet here we will offer you basic idea followed by a Free Video.

These ancient Chinese methods are extremely potent and will diminish your symptoms by 20-30% in first 21 days!

And any will agree, the best is that anyone can add these methods in to daily routine without much trouble and pain since it can take only 12 -15 minutes of time. About that, we will give you all details in later chapters - this ancient Qigong routine we present in book will simply surprise you, by its simplicity and powerful potency.

Many people have tried to 'alter' different complex therapies in order to make them easier and manageable. The book is intended to help celiac, individuals suffering from gluten intolerance along with their families. It is huge help to manage daily routine and diet with simple purpose to assist one in living a normal, comfortable and healthy gluten free lifestyle. For many, this guide will in fact present the bright light on the end of a dark tunnel.

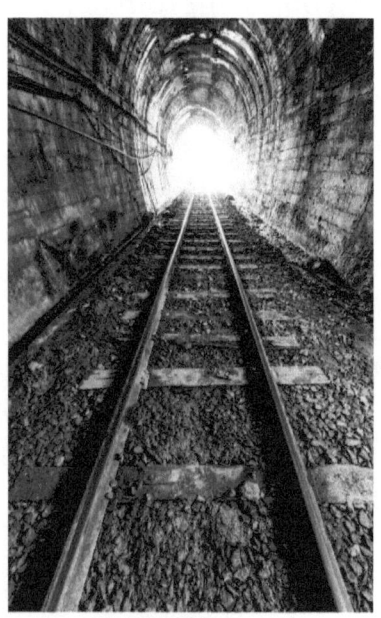

Who May Use This Book?

This book is recommended for:

-        Anyone experiencing celiac disease symptoms
-        Individuals suffering from any sort of gluten allergy or gluten intolerance
-        For those not sure what is wrong, but suffer from symptoms resembling sensitivity to gluten
-        Dietitians and Nutritionists that seek effective methods and remedies for their clients
-        Physicians and nurses
-        Family members of the person that is affected by gluten intolerance and / or celiac disorder
-        Restaurant and Hotel businesses personal and management (as well as Chefs, owners and anyone else in business of serving food to people)

This book features different useful advice; suggestions as well as ideas that will help you improve overall health and quality of life.

Best Way to Use This Guide

This book should be considered to be support to and alternative to classical medical approach. Best is, off course, to find reliable dietitian and/or a physician, who is specialized in gluten-free conditions, diet and celiac disease. The book is best to be used as a guide or complement to the experts' instructions.

This book is published with aims to:

-Increase awareness of gluten allergies

-Help you with better understanding of gluten allergies, gluten intolerances and celiac disease.
-Explain major differences between those conditions

-Offer you *simple, effective method for healing of the immune system,* that will by huge % help and possibly cure you from the gluten intolerance or allergy to gluten.

-Clearly explain symptoms and complications related to celiac disease and gluten intolerance

-Introduce you to a proper diagnosis, blood testing etc.

-Teach you about safe/dangerous ingredients in gluten-free food

-Share practical tips on staying safe while eating out

-Inspire and assist you in cooking various gluten-free dishes

This is a step-by-step guide to learn everything you really need to know about gluten intolerance related problems and the ways to prevent them for a long term effortlessly.

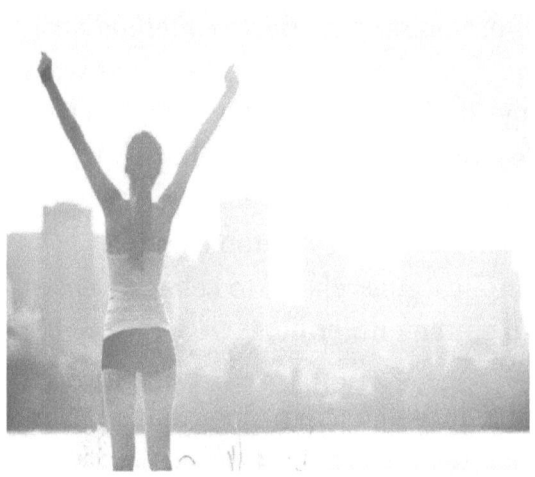

INTRODUCTION

A large number of people have been facing difficulties caused by adverse reaction to gluten, especially in the western countries. Some claim that it is due to bad eating habits, i.e. over consumption of baked goods, bread and processed foods. In essence, it can be described very fast so it looks easy and simple.

When our immune system is developing in childhood, our bodies were not totally familiar to antigens. Some authors in a field explain that is the reason due to which gluten has been considered by our immune system to be allergen or interloper. Reality is little more complex than that.

When it comes to gluten and gluten related health issues, basically three different types of diagnoses exist - gluten sensitivity, gluten intolerance and celiac disease. They naturally have different symptoms and indications. One of the biggest mistake person can make, is to count on Internet based information, magazines and unreliable info products related to these health issues.

Not as tragic but not totally helpful and incomplete approach is to focus only on external aspects – diet, recipes, cookbooks etc.

Good diet is important but possibility of re-rebuilding auto immune system is not for neglecting as well, isn't it? Another thing: some of the books (just like this one) can help and those that are good will benefit you for sure yet, you have to get a professional opinion from a medical professional. Yes, we know it is not always easy to get a reliable doctor and in that quite few complications are included. However, our honest advice (based on years of experience) is that, you should get accurate diagnosis from the specialist. There is nothing better you can do in the beginning. Instead of relying on self-diagnosis, do your self a favor and get diagnosed properly. In that way, you will know 'where are you at'. Next most important answers you need to get, depend on that – a lot about 'what you should do' you will be able to read right here in this guide.

Again, Celiac disease is an autoimmune disorder in which the body of the person cannot tolerate the grain proteins and foods made of certain grains like wheat, barley, rye, etc. in which gluten is found. Oats have always been included in the 'forbidden' list, together with grains. Few of more recent studies prove that, if consumed in moderation, oats are safe for healthy adults and children who are on gluten-free diet. Studies are still needed to find out the long-term contamination and safety issues. Hence, oats are not yet recommended in that sense, at least not in Canada and the US celiac organizations. One more fact that we have to know is that gluten intolerance as well as celiac disorder was once considered rare, but it nowadays became the prevalent in the western world countries, especially in US.

You will read or hear that following 100% Gluten-Free diet strictly is the only sure-shot treatment for this life-long disorder. There is a lot of truth to that and it is naturally the path one has to follow when faced with the gluten related health issues. In this book however you get to another aspect of the inner treatment that is effective and practical.

When you suffer from a painful condition, off course the first thing you do is to extinguish it. Better however is to know exactly why that occurred and solve that cause, so that pain and discomfort won't re-appear.

It is not so entirely easy to follow an ideal gluten-free diet, but it has to be done. That will help you avoid the symptoms and complications related to the disorder. In order to manage diet and lifestyle, people diagnosed with celiac disease or gluten intolerance should seek help and start reorganizing necessary elements and aspects of life in a right way.

In this book, we have tried our best to provide you with all needed practical information not only to get started but also to remain gluten free but happy and satisfied.

CHAPTER 1

What is Celiac Disease?

Also known as Gluten-Sensitive Enteropathy or Celiac Sprue, Celiac Disease is severe autoimmune and digestive disease, which damages the lining of small intestine when gluten foods are eaten.

Gluten is a kind of protein, which is mostly found in various types of grains. Whole issue with gluten intolerance and especially Celiac it is in suffering from intestinal damage – by time (and often within quite short time period) it becomes difficult to absorb vital nutrients from food. Digestive process simply fails (in some percentage or totally) to absorb needed and very important nutrients such as calcium, fat, folate and iron.

According to the estimates, around one in a hundred of people actually has celiac disease, though only few have been diagnosed. In 2001 for example, the average age of individual suffering from this disease was around 45 years. Earlier during 80's and before, celiac disease was considered to be pretty much a childhood disease.

Now often, medical personal tends to disregard the fact that it is not important if individual currently suffers from symptoms of. Sometimes, the person may feel healthy and the symptoms of the disease just suddenly appear. How is that? We guess it is interesting to know more about it.

You already know that Celiac disease is a serious disorder of autoimmune system that causes damage to the small intestine's lining. Due to this damage, our body finds it difficult to absorb gluten in complete and much needed way. Off course, the simplest conclusion we all get is that in order to control and avoid the health problems, the best is to avoid gluten-based foods in diet. Off course, there is more to this. If you will allow us to get bit of philosophical, and quote an ancient eastern proverb that pretty much explains the problem with approach of modern medicine:

"If you want tree in your backyard to grow, you need to nurture its root. Watering the branches, flowers, fruits or trunk of a tree is not going to help..."

It's common sense and it has already been established that anyone, especially individual with developed symptoms, has to avoid Gluten based food. Nevertheless one has to approach the root cause of gluten intolerance disorder. Sometimes, "has to", "must" and similar terms are just too authoritative and we normally avoid using them – in this case however, importance of getting deeper understanding is so huge that we sort of feel confortable when saying:

'If you want to get healthy and live full life, you simply must address the roots of the problem!'

Keep in mind that Celiac Disease is not what most people think – an allergy. *You might not be allergic to gluten – that is really important to keep in mind.* That would mean it is possible to eat different type of food containing grains with gluten, such as barley, rice or wheat. But when celiac disease grows, the gluten intolerance occurs and it is most likely to take other forms.

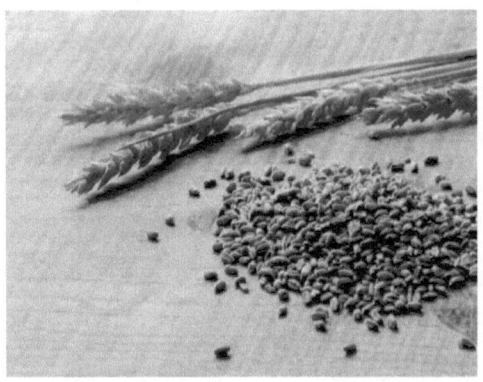

Now, the other way around is also IMPORTANT fact and many people (as well as some experts in a field) are confused about this. In that way the confusion and misunderstanding is getting spread further. Please understand that on the other side, having gluten intolerance _doesn't necessarily mean you have celiac disease_. Some people just don't! Issue here is simple: you have to know ☺ . One simply has to be sure exactly what your current condition is. Determination of having typical or critical symptoms is not enough profound and it is way from being reliable "method".

In some man, women and also children, celiac disease is diagnosed only when they undergo the proper and reliable medical testing. These individuals are just capable of eating things that contain gluten without suffering many or hardly any noticeable and disturbing symptoms.

1.1   Symptoms of Celiac Disease

The biggest issue with celiac disease is that it has wide range & number of symptoms. Many times that is confusing its self. One thing before heading to symptoms: let's explore the causes of celiac disease a bit. We won't make it long or complicated to understand, that's a promise. We are (most of us are) just tired of long, theoretical approaches that do nothing but spend our time, without really helping us.

In shortest – we all (should) know, immune system of our body is designed to prevent and defend our system from 'alien' invaders. When the individual suffering from celiac disease consumes gluten-based food, their immune system produces antibodies that are meant to 'fight and defend' the body from gluten. It however does more - it attacks the intestinal lining of digestive system as well. With this problem happening, the intestines of a person get affected and basically get inflamed. The hair-like structures or "villi" placed all over the small intestine's lining get damaged because of this. The Villi is responsible for absorbing the nutrients from gluten-based food. When these structures are damaged, body isn't able to digest the nutrients entirely and that's how one is left malnourished. As time passes, destructive nature of this catches on.

It doesn't matter how much you eat, amount of food isn't important – what you eat and how your body reacts to what you eat is crucial point. You see the problem bit differently?

One of the most common (and unfortunately often times not taken seriously) signs of celiac disease is the fatigue – feeling of having no (not enough) energy, weakness. Type of the fatigue that person experiences has the same cause yet how person perceives it is different, simply because we are not all the same. Different lifestyle, eating and sleeping habits, cleanliness and mental state as well as various other details of life, simply create different type of 'impression' of basically same thing.

How the lack of energy and fatigue hits you and changes the life routine maybe 'different' in practically each and every individual.

And yet, related to gluten intolerance and celiac disorder, there is ONE and ONLY cause of the fatigue. Problem majority people run in to is in the (already addressed) approach of the modern western medicine. If you think about this with open mindset, you will easily understand how risky, shallow and inefficient that is. Let us be even more specific about this:

For example, the nutritionists or medical specialist will use words like this:

"The fatigue you feel, occurs due to poor ability to absorb iron and few other nutrients..."

Is that true? YES, it is – what is the problem you may ask at this point.

Well, *problem is right there*. If we do not have full understanding of how and why this is happening we cannot prevent it and what to speak about going direction healing gluten intolerance disorder. Real problem is *NOT in the symptoms* of celiac but how we understand and deal with the symptoms. Off course, we have to understand what are clear and sure indications of celiac or other types of gluten intolerance.

For that reason, let's continue. Establishing (chronic) fatigue as a common symptom, there exist wide range of other symptoms; some of them often cause the misdiagnosis. It is common fact that not everyone is able to detect all the symptoms manifested. Here is a list of some of the possible symptoms you should be aware of:

-Digesting issues, such as stomachache, bloating, gas, pale stool, diarrhea and sudden weight loss

-Low blood count (Iron Deficiency, popularly called Anemia)
-Seizures not connected to other apparent cause

-Growth and developing issues in children

-Muscle cramps, bone / joint pain and other related musculoskeletal problems

-Missed monthly periods in women

-Sores in mouth (Aphthous Ulcers)

-Tingling sensation in legs (due to low calcium presence and nerve damage)

-Depression (amazingly enough but yes, it can be directly relevant to Gluten intolerance disorder)

-Vomiting

-Nausea

-Hair fall or losses of hair quality just like thinning, breaking of the hair etc.

These are the common symptoms and in our opinion and experience enough to know about. According to estimates, there are around 250 variations of celiac and gluten intolerance symptoms but going in that detailed listing isn't the goal of this guide and it won't really help you out. Why? It is explained previously but it is important and so allow us to repeat that line, it will benefit all readers:

"Real problem is NOT in (knowing all - all about) the symptoms but how we understand and deal with what causes the

problems (and the symptoms) within your body".

Right there is the point and the direction we take to within *Happy & Gluten Free Lifestyle Guide*. Instead of losing time, money and the nerves on the huge list of symptoms, combinations of those symptoms and analyzing them, we prefer to address the essence of the problem and offer you practical & easy to follow tips as well as possible solutions. Not just any solutions but those that hit hard, exactly at root cause of these health disorders.

1.2   Crucial Mistake of Western Medicine

Probably most important this we would like you to know at this moment is, you don't need to worry and be in stress. You can definitely ease up your health situation, avoid discomfort and pain and live a happy a sound life. You can heal your gluten intolerance and most probably celiac disease as well.

But, as a best start, you have to be sure about what's actually going on within your body. In order to do that, there are simply few things we suggest and you should think about them seriously. You may find another logical step to what you have to achieve but if you simply follow these steps, diagnosis part of the equation is going to be cleared:

1) Go through a normal blood test – arrange for looking after the antibodies that are related to this disease. You may save a ton of time and energy with this simple blood test.

2) In case your test results are found positive, you probably should arrange for small intestine's biopsy. In this test, the villi are analyzed and in order to do so, professionals in a laboratory or doctors office will take

a small sample of the tissue. The villi are analyzed in depth – level of damage or signs and type of damage is what professionals are going to look for.

3)   Now, if your biopsy test results come back as positive, it's time to take (or continue with) steps towards the healing, starting with clean gluten-free diet.

As earlier indicated, the popular western "outside" approach is not even near to anything person may consider as complete. I know we are sort of repetitive about this but you see, in today's modern society we are strongly influenced by that very mindset (in our home and family, school, university and any other form of education as well as trough mass media, internet, etc. etc.)

Lets clear up one more thing right now: we are NOT saying 'everything we get from modern medicine and western approach to health is bad and useless'. What we are saying is that in case of many health conditions, including celiac it's way too less. We need to know more, see the things in much 'wider angle' and yet deal only with practices that are beneficial and effective. In short...

...Always keep in mind we want to heal the root causes of the problem – NOT the external contra indication of the problem.

Going towards the process and practices of complete healing will offer you a lot – especially if you decide to take the advantage of this lifestyle guide. You will be assisted, inspired and supported in various ways throughout this work and that will lead you to fast improvement and healing of your body.

For example, good diet will improve your condition; symptoms and discomforts will stop appearing and make you feel much better. Avoiding gluten is major part of the complete approach to treatment of celiac disease.

In addition, here described ancient Qigong routine will generate a healthy energy flow throughout your body and so boost up your energy levels in all aspects. Healthy and increased energy flow will (over the short time frame) heal everything you need to get 'repaired' and healed within your body. If you continue with that practice, your autoimmune system disorder will be eventually become healed and you won't have to seek any further help , treatment of medicine.

1.3   Health Complications Related to Celiac Disease

This part of our Happy & Gluten Free Lifestyle Guide is basically here in order to further stimulate your decision of moving towards solution and effective healing, regardless of what type of gluten intolerance you suffer from and how severe your condition currently is. Bellow listed health issues are not pleasant but it is needed to know about them. Due to celiac disease, one is likely to face health conditions and problems such as:

- Infertility or miscarriage
- *Osteoporosis*– occurs due to lack of vitamin D and calcium.
- Neutral Tube defects and other birth defects with newborn, all due to poor digestion of folic acid and other vital nutrients.
- Thyroid gland related problems
- Lupus
- Type 1 Diabetes
- Rheumatoid arthritis

1.4   Getting Diagnosed

We did touch this matter and yet, let's go fast over few aspects of it. If you are going to be checked at credible medical center, your doctor will conduct a thorough physical checkup and ask different questions about your medical history. Along with conducting blood test(s) in order to detect what specific type of antibodies related to celiac disease you may suffer from, your physician will also conduct other types of tests in order to find out the symptoms of nutritional deficiencies, such as low iron levels (which are directly responsible for developing an anemia).

While being diagnosed, you may be also asked to give sample of stool – medical personal will need to analyze it for fat because in celiac disease, the bodies digestive processes fail to absorb the fat from food. In addition, you will also have to be tested by a biopsy. To conduct biopsy, an endoscope is inserted into small intestine through mouth in order to detect damage to the villi. That process isn't confortable at all – many do a fatal mistake of NOT going trough it. If you want our honest advice, you need to go through it and only so, you will be sure where you at. Once you get the results back you will know – simple as that.

If anyhow possible, please try to approach a doctor's office or medical professional that recognizes or maybe even supports the holistic forms of medicine but DO NOT (and we really mean it) please don't approach any unreliable medical office or laboratory. This is very important; you have to get a solid and definitive, sure diagnosis.

1.5   Treatment from 'Outside'

Simple! If you are diagnosed with celiac disease, you (most probably) cannot eat foods that contain gluten, such as wheat, oats, barley etc. Avoiding gluten will improve your health condition and remove suffering due to indications of celiac disease.

Most of the medical professionals will tell you something like:

"Dear Sir / Madam, you will simply have to live without eating anything containing gluten for the rest of your life".

And yet, that isn't necessarily the fact! For many modern man and woman that suffer from gluten intolerance that is a fact. However, this is neither a definite thing nor it is reality for everyone due to following:

1) Please understand - you can be healed, you can become free of Celiac and Gluten intolerance – condition you are in now are NOT your destiny. There is a way out!

2) Some individuals diagnosed with celiac disease have severe damage to the intestine, which cannot be healed quite easily, quickly and sometimes completely. Such patients may need strong food supplements and special medically

recommended procedures. But, hope is always there! Taking to both aspects presented in this guide, gluten-free diet and energy systems recovery is needed..

The way out is simply not only hidden within the external approach to treatment. The solution is actually in effective ways to bettering the immune and autoimmune system of the body. What we are sure about will work for you is the ancient Qigong practice we will present it in later chapters. Important for now is to accept the fact that, before you heal the root cause of your disorder, you need to maintain the gluten free diet and life style. If you start eating gluten-based food again, the problems will re-appear.

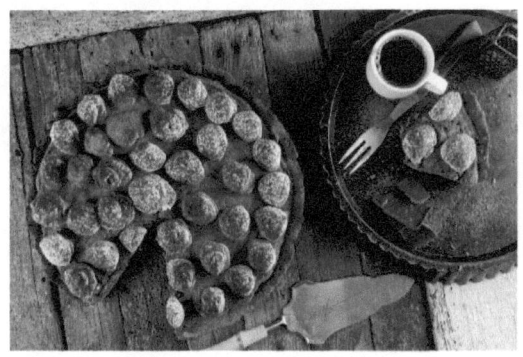

Gluten Free Lifestyle

Gluten-free diet can add a major change in your lifestyle. You have to change your eating pattern, such as what you choose for your daily meals, for parties or for your Sunday brunch. Going gluten-free means you have to avoid several dietary foods, such as cereals, pasta, and processed foods, which contain gluten. If you are buying packaged foods, you have to take extra care and prevent shopping the foods and products that have gluten. Read the label of packaged foods before buying. If you are eating at restaurant, consider reading ingredients and ask about it before you order. That is common sense, right?

Suffering celiac disease doesn't mean that tasty and enjoyable dishes are not going to be the part of your reality. Well-balanced diet is what you need. Here are few simple guidelines you may like to consider:

- You can eat pasta and breads made from ingredients other than gluten
- Eat fresh foods
- Do not eat artificially processed food
- Eat fresh vegetables, fruits and nuts
- Avoid fish and meats not because they contain gluten but because they are very heavy for digestion and are bad for you overall health and recovery.
- Ask your nutrition expert or dietitian that specializes in nutrition

and food, about details of gluten-free diet.
- Explore and find recipes that suit you, your lifestyle and situation
- Avoid stagnant and monotone diet plans and habits

CHAPTER 2

The Basics of Gluten Free Diets

Nowadays, a large population of the world has been suffering from celiac disease. When it comes to gluten sensitivity, one question pops out; is our body is structured to consume grains? Around 10000 years ago, grains were not the part of daily diet because they were not cultivated. In pre-agricultural era, people didn't suffer from several digestive and metabolic diseases, which have been related to eating processed foods and grains like cereals, pastries, breads and other new-age delights.

Within few decades, the cases of type 2 diabetes, metabolic syndrome, obesity and other disorders have been dramatically increased. Hence, gluten-free diet has been widely recommended for those who have been suffering from gluten sensitivity or celiac disease.

2.1 What is Gluten? Why Is It 'Bad'?

Gluten is, generally, a type of protein found in grains such as barley, triticale and wheat of all types. Gluten adds the elasticity, giving shape to food grains. Its role is to glue the substances, just like regular glue that keeps things together. Gluten is also used in hair products, cosmetics, and other dermatological products. It is mainly found in wheat, rye and barley (wheat is found in pasta, breads, baked items, soups, sauces, pasta, roux, and salad dressings; barley is found in soups, malt, beer, food coloring, and malt sugar; and rye in cereals and rye bread).

Why is Gluten Bad for Your Health?

Over the past couple of years, awareness in relation to the ill effects of gluten-based food has been increased. According to a 2013 survey, around 1/3rdof population in US is actively skipping gluten from their daily diet. Several studies prove that gluten is harmful for our body. Here are some reasons why person should be determent to avoid it:

Celiac Disease (Often) Remains Undetected

Gluten mainly has two types of protein– gluten in and gliadin. Gliadin is normally responsible for negative effects in humans. When you make the dough with water and flour, gluten adds elasticity with sticky links of proteins on the dough and bread rises when it is baked. The glue-like properties are the ones from which the word "gluten" derives. When immune system is exposed to gluten after it accesses the digestive tracks, it is by mistake misunderstood for 'attack' on the body. Due to weakness and exposure to few different conditions, gliadin is perceived like a substance coming from destructive elements and outside invaders, like the bacteria. That is the simplest way to explain what is actually going on.

When gluten sensitivity goes severe, it causes celiac disease. In this condition, gluten proteins in our digestive system are attacked by the immune system. Due to the exposure of gluten, the immune system attacks both intestinal wall and gluten. Hence, celiac disease is considered as autoimmune disorder. Due to immune reaction, the intestinal wall is degenerated and it over the time causes lack of sufficient nutrients, anemia, digestive problems, failure to thrive, fatigue and higher % of fatal diseases risk.

The recent studies show that around 80% of individuals don't even know that they are suffering from celiac disease or its early stages. Currently, around 1.5% of the world population is suffering from celiac disease, and it is increasing.

Gluten Sensitivity vs. Celiac Disease

If you are suffering due to negative reactions connected to gluten, celiac disease is not necessarily the cause of your trouble. **Gluten Intolerance** or **Gluten Sensitivity** is another common problem. Even though gluten sensitivity cannot be clearly defined, it literally refers to having some kind of serious negative reactions to gluten.

Point in simple words is that many of us may have non-celiac gluten intolerance – simply, if you are facing negative reactions caused by gluten, you may not have developed celiac disease. Another word, if that is the case, your immune system won't attack your own inner tissues in order to 'auto-defend'. Several symptoms are identical with the developed celiac disease, such as:

- Stomachache
- Bloating
- Diarrhea
- Fatigue and
- Pain in joints / bones.

All in all, gluten intolerance is a lot more widespread than celiac disease, and also causes several adverse effects. And the irony is that there is no proper way to diagnose it.

Gluten Causes Serious Effects, Even You Don't Suffer from Gluten Sensitivity

In some studies, people who didn't have celiac disease and never diagnosed with any gluten intolerance, still had serious reactions to gluten.

Around 30 individuals who have ill-tempered bowel syndrome were recommended to either have gluten free or gluten-based diet. Those who had gluten-based food had more bloating, pain, fatigue and inconsistent stool, as compared to others who didn't.

According to other studies, gluten is also responsible to cause inflammation in small intestine and degenerate intestinal lining. Due to gluten, a barrier is created on the intestine due to which unwanted elements are leaked through the blood stream. There are several other digestive problems caused due to irritable bowel syndrome (IBS). Around 14% of US residents are afflicted with IBS.

Brain Disorders Related to Gluten

Well, you may perceive these lines as scary but unfortunately this is nothing but a fact. For example, even though gluten intolerance disorders basically affect the gut, they can also cause serious brain disorders. Gluten consumption is responsible to several neurological issues. It is known as *Gluten-Sensitive Idiopathic Neuropathy*.

In a study that was conducted on patients who had various brain illnesses, 30 out of 53 patients had antibodies fighting the gluten present in the blood. **Cerebellar Ataxia** is found to be the major neurological illness, which is considered to have relation with gluten intolerance. It is a serious illness, which makes the patient unable to move, keep the balance and even to talk.

Several cases of this disease are directly connected to consumption of gluten. Cerebral ataxia causes irreversible damage to the "Cerebellum", part of brain that plays important role in control of motoric functions of the nervous system.

According to some studies, there is a strong connection between gluten sensitivity, gluten consumption and cerebellar ataxia. A controlled trial has been made on patients who were improved dramatically with gluten-free diet. Interestingly enough, gluten-free diet is also helpful to control several other brain disorders like Schizophrenia, Epilepsy and Autism.

2.2 Getting Started with Gluten-Free Diet

On the start, just like if your doctor recommends you avoiding gluten from your diet you may feel little worried. That is totally OK and natural since Gluten based ingredients are probably the solid part of your diet. Foods just like pizza, pasta, beer, hamburgers, crackers, sandwiches and breads have gluten and they are naturally big "no-no" when it comes to adopting clean gluten-free diet.

At first, it may seem pretty challenging. Adopting new diet plan is not easy for most of us in the beginning. All you need to understand the value of the naturally gluten-free foods vs. range of gluten-free packaged products in supermarkets. After that, you can in fact life comfortably a clean Gluten free lifestyle.

When you start with clean gluten-free and natural food based diet, first few weeks you will experience a change and will benefit you more and more. Once you start feeling the benefits, you will easily and automatically incline toward gluten-free variants of breads and other food items in the market. Make sure not to 'blindly' buy and overly consume just any products carrying gluten-free label: gluten-free cakes, snacks and cookies still have sugar and calories and they may not provide proper nutrition.

Also check the food supplements and medicine you are using. Also, while eating out, ask for gluten-free menu; nowadays in the restaurants it becomes easier to get one. If not available, ask the chef or the restaurant personal in order to make sure the meal you have ordered is gluten free and safe for you.

If you belong to the family where only you have to stick to gluten-free food, beware of the cross contamination. Keep your cooking equipment and utensils separately. Don't share condiments – even a piece of bread that contains gluten (for example in the peanut butter) can cause negative effects in your body and recreate negative chemical / autoimmune reactions.

2.3 Who Should and Shouldn't Live a Gluten-Free Life?

One thing many people misunderstood is losing weight. Gluten-free diet is not recommended for weight loss. It solely treats people who suffer from gluten intolerance disorders and celiac disease. One has to keep in mind that gluten is a protein, present in various healthy and whole-grain foods that are all rich sources of vital nutrients and fiber.

If you start gluten-free diet just to lose weight, you will actually cause damage to your body. According to the 2010 Dietary Guidelines of US national dieting guide, we should eat at least 14g of fiber for consuming every 1000 calories. This way, we should consume at least 25 to 35 grams per day. Fiber keeps heart healthy and makes us feel fuller. Hence, we should maintain balance between consumption of calories and fiber. That's clear.

As you already know, Celiac disease causes damage to small intestine and makes it unable to absorb nutrients from healthy food. It causes reaction and makes immune system to act against gluten – that is found in cereals, barley, wheat, oats and rye. If you are diagnosed with this disease, your doctor will recommend you to avoid consuming foods, which may have gluten, especially whole grain ones.

2.4 Checking Food Label

For getting started with gluten-free food, you have to learn and master this skill. Reading food label in proper and safe way is a skill mainly because of expert ways food manufacturers use to hide certain facts. We all are familiar with those tiny printed labels. Now, this is really more important for you and your well-being. Check out the label of each food product you pick from the shelves of supermarket. Even if the package mentions "Gluten-Free", the product recipes vary. So, check the label of all products.

Depending where you live, you may have different conditions. In US as of August 2014, product labels stating "Gluten Free" should adhere to FDA regulations. It became voluntary to use this label. But in same time, some gluten-free / safe foods may not use it. We should read the labels of dressings, soups, and sauces carefully because most of them have gluten hidden as wheat starch. If you find "Brewer's yeast", "rye", "barley" or "Malt" on the label, don't buy the food because it is not safe for you. Soy sauce is fermented with wheat. So, it also contains gluten.

Having "Wheat Free" product doesn't mean that it is gluten-free. It may have rye or barley that can adversely affect your body if you have gluten sensitivity.

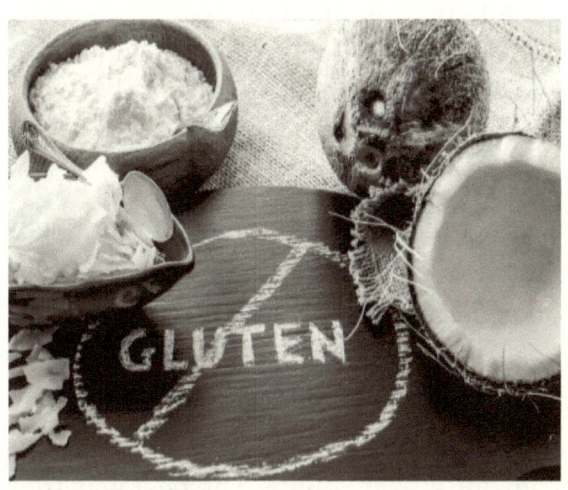

2.5 Foods to Adopt and to Avoid in Gluten-Free Diet

First of all, you have to throw out all the doubtful foods from your pantry and restock with those foods that are naturally gluten-free. All the plain and fresh vegetables and fruits are naturally gluten-free. You have to be wary with dressings, breading and sauces.

All seasoned and unprocessed protein foods are gluten-free. Processed foods like pizza, hamburgers, pasta etc. may or may not have gluten, according to the ingredients and brand. Several starches and grains are gluten-free, such as rice, corn, millet, quinoa and potatoes. Choose only unprocessed versions of such foods because processed ones like crackers, chips and tortillas have gluten-based ingredients. Gluten-free oats are basically safe for people who are suffering from gluten-sensitivity. The best way to go gluten-free is to avoid beverages and foods, which have bulgur, barley, graham flour, farina, rye, wheat, spelt, triticale, and semolina and matzo meal.

Simple as that!

CHAPTER 3

The Health Benefits of Gluten-Free Diet

Getting started with gluten-free diet is (in our opinion) for most man and women a big deal. One has lot new things to deal with and learn. We face a lot of mental hurdles. But these challenges are definitely worth the effort. If you think your body reacts adversely to gluten, it's time to start testing out gluten-free diet and therefore end the migraines, poor digestion, pain, itchy skin, arthritis, etc.

In this chapter, we are going to focus the things we must expect from gluten-free diet. Before that, let's go over the health benefits of gluten-free diet.

Health Benefits of Gluten-Free Diet

Efficient 'Cure' for All Kind of Stomach Problems

If you have celiac disease and you are facing digestive issues, you should start gluten-free diet. There are many people who face sensitivity to dairy products and have pollen and wheat allergies. It may also cause some of the symptoms related to gluten intolerance, but gluten-free diet can resolve pretty much all these problems. If you combine clean diet habits with Qigong practice and / or meditation, you actually have a winning formula in your hands. It needs time and persistence but it is worthy of every second or your time.

Improved Brain Functions

Eliminating gluten from your diet may help you improve your focus, mood and 'clear thinking' ability. People who have gluten intolerance are reported to have 'foggy' focus and thinking, headaches, depression and symptoms like ADHD, according to the reports of National Foundation for Celiac Awareness. The brain faces certain side effects, which are related to inflammation molecule of certain kind known as cytokines. This molecule is released when person with gluten sensitivity consumes gluten. These cytokines are related to brain function.

Improved Energy Level

If you have gluten sensitivity, there are chances that you are feeling problem is absorbing minerals and vitamins. Due to this malnutrition, you may be facing reduced energy levels and feeling tired. People who have sensitivity to gluten may have been facing overall tiredness and weakness. Anemia also causes fatigue and prevents absorption of iron because of inflammation in intestine. Avoiding gluten may be something you need (even without suffering from Gluten intolerance) in order to enhance energy level and power of your focus and attention.

Reduces Inflammation

Inflammation is mainly caused due to cytokines that have strong negative affect to body tissues. People who have gluten sensitivity may also suffer from muscle cramping, joint paint and numb legs. Due to chronic inflammation, you might have weak health, pain and even some of the serious and deadly diseases such as cancer. Gluten intolerance may also cause itchy rashes and inflammation of skin tissues. By avoiding gluten, you will experience improved skin condition.

Success Stories

We have many, literally hundreds and thousands of similar testimonials, emails and experiences. In case you need to hear few, take a minute and read trough these:

Speech Delay Recovered by Gluten-Free Diet

> *"I tried gluten-free diet on one of my kids. He used to say only a few words regularly by the age of 3 years and he communicated mostly with his gestures. He was thriving but at very slow rate. On the other side, his younger sister was growing normally. On his third birthday, I took a resolution to give him casein-free and gluten-free food for two weeks. Just a few days later, he started talking rapidly. It was the gluten which causing problem in his physical and mental ability. Once I removed gluten from his diet, he started recovering his ability to exploring words. Each*

day, he picks a new word. After nine months without gluten, he greatly improved his verbal skills."

- ***Lauren, Ca***

Gluten-Free Diet Reduces Depression

"In our daily lives, we are used to eat gluten, more often than not. I often feel the effects of depression with more intensity. Sometime, I feel "emotional heaviness" which was another troublesome problem. My physician recommended me to start gluten-free diet. Now, I don't have to face such kind of emotional weakness and depression every day. "

- ***Daniel, LA***

What to Expect from Gluten-Free Food?

If you are preparing for any significant change in life, you should know what to expect beforehand. At the beginning, it is going to be a major 'joy-killer'. You may even have to face a huge emotional crisis in the beginning. But such emotions are just a short phase that will soon melt away and become the past!

You are about to go on board with a major lifestyle change. So, it is important to know what challenges are waiting for you on your path. Here's what you should expect to have in your gluten-free diet regimen.

You Might Make Few Mistakes

First of all, you are about to learn several new things about baking, cooking, and shopping groceries within few weeks or months. So, you may not get everything right in the first move, which is just normal thing to expect. If you keep learning every day, you will be exceptional in getting 100% gluten free and safe within short time.

Don't Expect Instant Results

Some of you may want to see instant improvements for which you have avoided gluten from your diet. Your body may need time to repair and heal. The condition you are in wasn't developed over few days, week or months. It was grown in to over the years and despite the potency of everything we share with you, some natural recovery healing time has to be there. You should monitor your body properly and expect to take time for healing. You won't face any trouble by avoiding gluten. So, before you make any decision, be prepared to give time to your bodily systems to heal.

Take Time to Learn

You have to take time to feed your body perfectly so it can be healthy.

Especially, your baking, cooking and shopping grocery may take longer time than usually for the first time. All you need to make room to go gluten free in your life. You can find less stress in transition if you take time to learn and to do it well.

Resistance

Most of us don't like any kind of change in our lives and environment. So, you should try to expect some adverse reactions. Gluten free lifestyle and diet is not a 'regular' lifestyle and diet. It can in fact heal your body completely and it is really very amazing – once you stick to it, you will see, feel and enjoy its power. You should stick to it and give time to it to work. Please do that.

Learn Skipping a Meal

At some point of time, you may face the situation where the only choice is gluten-based food. You can either eat gluten or skip it. For several years, you have been eating gluten and you (most likely) were scared of skipping your meal. But from now on, you have to consider skipping a meal and learning to do it – nothing bad will happen. OPPOSITE is fact – you will get the power from that practice. You can drastically win over the fear of pain by skipping the meal. So, you can easily handle this problem without harming yourself.

Stay Prepared for Success

Most of us have low self-control as far as having tasty food is concerned. If you have wheat-based ingredients in your home, you are probably going to eat it. It is better to keep gluten away from your eyes. If cravings and temptations are your problem, get these things out of your kitchen. Just try everything to keep it away from your eyes. It's honest as well as simple!

Stay Up to Learn

Even though you know a lot about baking, you have to know a lot about gluten-free baking and cooking. Look for it as a bigger experiment and try to see what you are going to learn.

Take Stance to Enjoy Your Food

You will quickly learn that you enjoy the food you now have on your gluten-free regimen. You can take responsibility - it is possible for you. You have to draw attention to your diet; probably you have to ensure that you are eating safe food in restaurant and at home. Do some research on cooking and make your domestic budget so you can have more room to have gluten-free diet.

Verdict

Despite some 'depressing' points I have discussed in this chapter, you are about to feel better with gluten-free diet and such small irritating moments (that are the price for achieving great things) are worth of each and every moment of a 'struggle'.

We can significantly shorten al that uncomfortable adjusting periods by implementation of exercise that will start rejuvenating our energy system from within.

That will make the free Gluten free diet 2x, 3x and even 10+x more effective. That is the unique feature or this "inside out" approach to gluten free lifestyle.

CHAPTER 4

What Doctors Do NOT Want You to (Ever) Know...

"Inner" Healing for Gluten Intolerance

Here in this part of the manual, we are going to present you a crucial aspect of healing and trouble less, Gluten free lifestyle. Title of the chapter is NOT the trick meant for grabbing you attention – it is real, more real than most people can imagine. Without touching ideas of conspiracy theories and New World Order, we just have to conclude that it is in fact an absurd and tragic situation. There are simple yet effective methods for different health issues and conditions out there, but are not available for most in need. That knowledge is nowadays not easily reachable for those in need. With the power of Internet, this gets better and yet...

It's shocking to me (and probably most of you) to see how many people are totally misguided by false claims about getting fit and being healthy. You probably know already that powerful industrial lobbies own most of the media, pharmaceutical industry and sports nutrition market for example. In that way, they massively market and sell huge amount of vitamins, proteins, powders, drugs and pills under different labels.

All the misguided messages and avalanche of pharmaceutical and wellness/fitness marketing could get summed up in one sentence:

"Fitness and health comes from and it depends on outside factors."

Wrong, Wrong, WRONG! … And dangerous for everyone who believes in those claims.

You see, I don't mind that industry lobby magnates get richer and richer, if that's what they want to do. But it saddens me is to see an endless wave of illusion sold successfully to people. Believe me when I say...

...Most of today's approaches to healing, exercise and fitness are not at all healthy!

Why?

In short, the modern approaches and most of the medicine experts are aimed at the external aspects of the body ... cardiovascular system muscles, external symptoms of a disease etc.

What is wrong with that?

Well, a few things for starters. Our good health doesn't JUST depend on the heart, the muscles and the lungs. The healthy functioning of all organs in the body (kidneys, gall bladder, bladder, spleen, long & short intestine, etc.) directly provides us with good fitness level and health. NO health there = NO health at all! That means low energy, and a constant struggle with health. That is no way to achieve any decent fitness level, especially not in the long run.

In relation to that, (any type of) gluten intolerance is very hard or nearly impossible to overcome without proper cure of the energy flow in the body and between the internal organs. Another way of showing this principle is through the ancient practice of Chi Kung. What we will offer to all of you is the quick way to solve this problem. Off course, video isn't most complete way to learn about the profound practice of Qigong and for that reason we are offering you here a brief overview and on the end of this chapter you will be instructed about how to get the Video. Exercises shown and explained in detail within Sifu Lee's Total Chi Fitness book and we simply do not have time to do that here. What is important for you to know is that these simple stretching movements are aimed at reviving and maintaining a strong energy flow throughout our gross and subtle body.

Once healthy functioning of the internal organs has been achieved (supported by a lot of Chi and blood flow), we can start enjoying the benefits of total health and fitness in all eleven of our systems: cardiovascular, digestive, endocrine, lymphatic, immune, muscular, nervous, reproductive, respiratory, skeletal, and urinary. Now, I am sure you got interested, right?

Without having a healthy body on the inside, what is the point of talking about health, fitness, wellness and enjoying life? I hope you are with us on this. If you are and these words mean something to you, we know you will enjoy this book.

Proof is in the Pudding

Real value is not hidden in what

someone says or writes. It is all about (and always was) the *practical benefits and results we actually get*. In our experience, the reality of life today demands an approach with as much practicality and efficiency as possible. Next to the previously explained differences, efficiency is the most prominent quality of Chi-Fitness exercises. In the same way as when Sifu is teaching a seminar or a private class, in this book I focus on practicality and efficiency inside of a process. You will be provided with a tool that you can use efficiently any time you want. If you do use it, you will be able to generate the same results as thousands of other practitioners – almost without being able to help it. The system is simple yet powerful, and people who use it start feeling the change in a fairly short time period. We can promise you that!

It is NOT only for the Celiac and Gluten intolerance health issues. Please check out the list bellow. These are main

81

health issues that are treated and healed successfully with these simple exercises. By making your life Qi energy flow better trough out your body, limbs and organs you will influence many health disorders and conditions, just like was being done for thousands of years:

- Lack of energy
- Headache
- Difficulties in maintaining focus
- Feelings of physical weakness
- Mental weakness
- Need to boost your energy level
- Need to boost Sport performance
- Need to boost working performance
- Desire to boost weight loss results
- Need to improve detoxing results
- Suffering from chronic pain
- Allergies (including Gluten Intolerance)
- Difficulty enjoying life without painkillers and/or medication
- High or low blood pressure issues
- Suffering from a digestion disorders
- Need to accelerate healing from illness or surgery

\-   Desire to prevent the chronic "I am sick and tired" feeling
\-   Need to boost your libido and sex drive;

Now, everyone who had read my 5-Minute Chi Boost program will recognize this list of benefits. All are listed there as well. So, what is the difference between these two programs and why is that important for us?

 In order to explain this in detail I need more space and therefore I'll do it right below.

"5-Minute Boost" – "Total Chi Fitness": Difference

Here is the short answer: these are two separate programs. Both work well and help people. Like the content of a good electric razor, this is a total package meant for consistent home use, and the other is the smaller unit meant for traveling. Both are of superb quality, but one gets more done while the smaller one is easier to carry but must be used more frequently. Women might better understand example of pre-packaged hair dye; it works well to touch up color points, but getting a hair dye job done at a real salon will last for weeks longer.

The methods described in my first book, 5-Minute Chi Boost, are very effective, but you don't have to read them to benefit from this set of Qigong exercises.

Naturally, the acupressure techniques in 5-Minute Chi Boost are not the only healing exercises I teach. The reason for that is actually simple to understand. 5-Minute Chi Boost is a program that does exactly what it promises: boosts your Chi in matter of a few hours or days. Anyone who needs boost of energy and quick help will appreciate these methods. If you do like 5-Minute Chi Boost or similar acupressure routine, do it! There is nothing wrong in that – you will accelerate your energy cycles and quality of your life energy will increase.

Yet, in order to really start working on deep causes behind the Gluten intolerance and the blockages that is causing the autoimmune disorders, one needs more – the powerful meridian stretching routine. From there, the energy level of a busy practitioner only continues to increase. My first Kindle bestseller 5-Minute Chi Boost was needed and wanted in order to offer the shortest and most practical Qi boost program, so that people could generate the results really fast.

However, most people with Gluten intolerance troubles simply need to go deeper, with more profound practice. For that reason I recommend you to start with the Total Chi Fitness routine right away.

It is really interesting to read emails I get from people who take my books and use them in day-to-day life. The messages

I get from those readers are very similar to those I've received over the last two and half decades of teaching. I'm very happy to read all reactions from people that read my book's on Amazon Kindle. Many readers give the identical feedback of the attendees at my 5-Minute Chi Boost seminar, after practicing the simple system for a while.

For example:

"... I like the 5-Minute Chi Boost program. I get (such and such) benefit) when I do it. However, when I forget to do my 'cycle', my problems seems to reappear. Is there anything that has a longer lasting effect?

- "I feel much better but I want more. My health problems seem to be deep-rooted can you show us something 'stronger'?"

- "In your book and in your email you are talking about assistance that is stronger and can help us even more. Where I can *read more about that?"*

People ask this question in various ways, conditioned by a range of circumstances in life. A few years back, I received an 18-page letter that essentially elaborated on only one of these questions. My answer always has been and still is the same.

My answer is "Yes", but you have to use common sense. No one can expect an instant 'magical' solution for a problem or a set of problems that have bothered you for several years or even decades. In the same way as I teach my students, I invite you to further expand the power and potency of the traditional art of Chi Kung. This book outlines complete Chi Kung exercises that have helped people for thousands of years – no question about that. They will also help you if you do them correctly. The learning curve is short, normally one or two weeks. However, you will need to set aside more time for doing them – not just five – ten minutes. Not to worry, it doesn't take a lot more time! Once learned, you can complete one Total Chi Fitness exercise set in about 15 to 20 minutes, and there is no need to repeat the cycle more than once. However, since autoimmune disorder such Celiac disease and gluten intolerance requires serious attention, you will need to be consistent in your practicing.

As you can see in Video that you receive with our book, the Total Chi Fitness program is fairly simple to perform and easy to learn. This routine influences each and every energy channel of the body, and can generate results that the 5-Minute Chi Boost program can't really offer to most practitioners and or most of the time. The main differences or additional benefits of Total Chi Fitness exercises are:

-Direct and stronger impact on root cause of health problems

-Higher strength for disease prevention

-Longer lasting effects on subtle and physical body

Simply speaking, these Total Chi Fitness Exercises are more profound and have longer lasting effects than anything else you may start practicing. The simple methods rely on stimulating pressure points and particularly generating a strong flow of life energy. Total Chi Fitness does the same, but by treating all meridians and pressure points on the body = full body. Compering these 2 approaches, one isn't better than the other – they are simply two programs with the same goals but a different approach.

Both can help you and both can heal you. If you have more health problems or if you are serious about preventing weakness, disease, lack of focus, tiredness, headaches (or the other symptoms listed above), I definitely recommend that you learn and start applying this program. If you only need a quick energy boost, just

stick to methods described in the
previously described book.

Powerful Qigong Routine Video

If you are not online right now while
reading this book, you can always visit
this link later. Please be advised, there is
a necessary procedure, demanded due to
anti spam rules and regulations.

1)   First visit the link
http://eepurl.com/6JUtP and subscribe to
our list.
2)   Confirm your email address
3)   Please allow up to 1h for getting
the email with the link to the Total Chi
Fitness Video.
4)   If you do not see the Video after 1h,
please check all the inboxes. spam filters
etc. That usually solves a problem

Thank you.

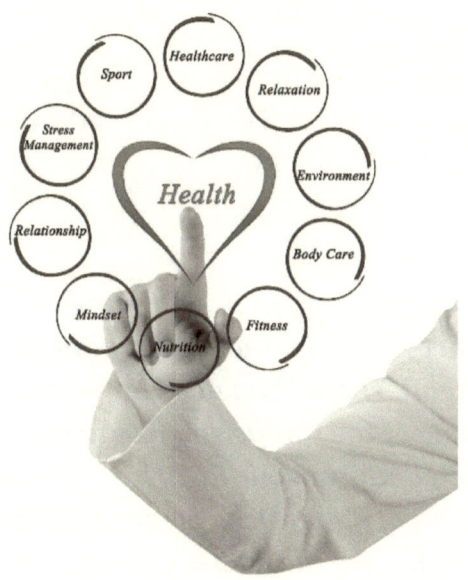

CHAPTER 5

Preparing Gluten-Free Meals Everyday

Planning gluten free-meals to kick-start your day is all about planning ahead. There is no need for giving up some of the things you like to eat. In fact, many of your favorite foods are made of gluten-free grains that taste exactly like the dishes you are obsessed with. You can make fantastically tasteful snacks easily as well as meals provided you have well-stocked kitchen.

If you are parent of a child with Celiac of gluten intolerance, or you cook for another person who has gluten-intolerance or celiac disease: before preparing meals, you should avoid the risks of cross contamination that is very important.

Have fresh fruits and vegetables, rice, corn, soy, and potato products. Don't choose flours made of rye, wheat, barley etc. Also avoid rolls, breads, cakes, breadcrumbs, croutons, pies, muffins, cookies, crackers, noodles, and cracker crumbs made of flours that contain gluten. Avoid sauces, soups, batters and gravies thickened with flours made of gluten.

5.1   Healthy Gluten-Free Breakfast Ideas to Kick-Start Your Day

There is no lack of healthy and delicious breakfast ideas for people who have celiac disease and gluten allergy. Hence, you won't end up feeling deprived. At first, the entire process of gluten-free diet may feel a bit disappointing. Lucky, there is no lack of hearty and healthy breakfast ideas to enjoy gluten free diet. Here are just some of the yummy breakfast options:

- **Gluten-Free Quinoa**–Whip up gluten-free bake, which contains cinnamon-spiced, soft apples; crispy almonds, and plump raisins. Bake apple-cinnamon batch before time to enjoy the healthy and delicious breakfast throughout the week.

- **Pumpkin Pie Muffins**–These fluffy and light muffins can be the delightful breakfast to kick-start your day. They are so sweet that you'll feel like a delight. They have around 140 Kcal per muffin. They will keep you feel full and satisfied throughout the morning.

- **Breakfast Polenta**–After intense morning workout, an instant bowl of polenta can give you the healthy dose of carbs, protein and comfort. It can easily be prepared (within 10 minutes) and an excellent vegetarian and gluten-free breakfast option for athletes who need instant meal for recovery.

- **Fresh Fruit Parfait** - It is yet another healthy and gluten-free breakfast option which can be enjoyed on the go. It is easy to make and is full of carbohydrates, protein, and healthy fats. It can keep you feel fuller for longer.

- **Banana Breads (Gluten-Free)** – This tasty, juicy breakfast staple can perk up your protein intake and fuel you up for an active day. Bananas make it more healthy and delightful. They are enriched with potassium to help ease bloating and water retention. You can grab your favorite loaf and have it on the go.

- **Gluten Free Pancakes** – Some people often want nothing more than pancakes for breakfast. If you are one of them, here is good news for you! You have no longer need to have a lot of wheat flour and buttermilk to prepare them. The recipe of making these amazing pancakes includes just honey, soymilk, buckwheat flour and almond and coconut oil so you can easily enjoy the taste of usual recipe without adding gluten.

- **Raw Banana Nutty Bars** – You can fulfill your half-day needs of vitamin E with 1 Oz. of raw banana nut bars. They can fulfill over 8% of your daily needs of calcium intake. You can enjoy an ideal gluten-free Sunday breakfast with this vegan and raw breakfast staple.

5.2   What to Pack on Your Gluten-Free Lunchbox?

As you see, adopting gluten-free diet doesn't mean you have to leave out your favorite muffins, biscuits, and pancakes. With bit of creativity and learning, you can keep enjoying the treats you "can't live without". Try these delicious and finger-licking gluten-free lunch recipes. Here are few ideas one can have for lunch meal:

- **GF Quinoa Salad –** Creamy and tasty Tahini dressing, this gluten-free Quinoa salad can be tastier than normal salads. For best cooking of quinoa, the quantity of water varies. So, be sure to read instructions on the package for getting the best results. Add toasted slivered almonds on the salad to get a twist.

- **Spicy Eggplant Lentil Salad –** You can make hot gluten-free and vegetarian salad by mixing lentils, eggplant and mangoes. You may choose from hot or medium variants of chili powders, salsa and curry powder to personalize its spiciness.

- **Hearty Gluten-Free Cheese Sandwich**–The no-knead, easy gluten-free bread has pleasing taste and great texture. You can enjoy warm bread slices with butter or make a healthy French toast or grilled tofu cheese sandwich.

- **Gluten-Free Biscuits made of Sorghum Flour**– Whether it is lunch, breakfast, or dinner, you can enjoy these biscuits with every meal. These biscuits get their traditional fluffy texture with naturally gluten-free Sorghum flour. You can enjoy oven-baked warm cookies with preserves and butter.

- **Asparagus Soup** – You can spice up this lemony garden-fresh soup with juicy red tomatoes, 'lite' coconut milk, and a touch of curry for added richness. It can be topped with plain yogurt or crème fraîche and served chilled or warm.

- **The Big-on-Taste Gluten-Free Juicy Oat Muffins**–These Gluten-Free fruity muffins can definitely entice those who don't have allergy with gluten. While preparing them, you can play along with fruits, by adding strawberries, dried blueberries, chopped apricots or raspberries. People who have celiac disease or gluten sensitivity shouldn't opt for nuts or dried fruit from bulk bins because they might be cross-contaminated with ingredients that contain gluten. So, it is wise to look for sealed containers.

- **Roasted Cauliflower Salad & Walnuts** – This roasted salad can be healthier with an earthy, irresistible sauce prepared with lemon, dill, tahini and walnuts. This roasted cauliflower salad can be served with pita and hummus.

5.3   Healthy Gluten Free Appetizers and Snack Ideas

If you are going to adopt gluten-free diet or strictly avoiding gluten from your diet, there are chances that you need to avoid wheat and dairy products as well.

At first, it may seem that you'll have nothing to eat. However in reality, the matter of fact is, you really can eat all sorts of satiating, healthy and nutritious meals. But first, let's clear out some of the important facts you should know.

Avoiding Milk and Dairy Products

If you have decided to avoid dairy products, remember that dairy product not only means milk. You have to eliminate milk products and the proteins based on milk, which are also added in many type of the processed food. You have to skip whey protein, kefir, yogurt, cream cheese, cheese, butter etc. Other packaged products contain casein and whey is also included because they are added in cereals, soups, chips, chocolate, dressings, protein snacks and snack bars.

Your gluten intolerance has nothing to do with your gluten-based foods; however it will greatly benefit your health if you can manage successfully avoiding milk and dairy-based products. The good thing about switching from normal to Gluten free diet is that you can easily adapt other habits without additional endeavor and sacrifice. This helpful advice you must likely take into consideration.

We have already explained, avoiding wheat doesn't really mean skipping all the diets that contains wheat, but adopting gluten-free diet means you have to avoid things that contains gluten in them. Gluten is mainly found in barley, wheat and rye. Traditional bread, pasta, foods that have fried coatings, rolls, pizza, noodles and beers also contains gluten. A lot of processed foods armada ingredients that contain gluten includes wheat flour, wheat starch, wheat berries, barley malt syrup, semolina, durum, graham, spelt, triticale etc. etc.

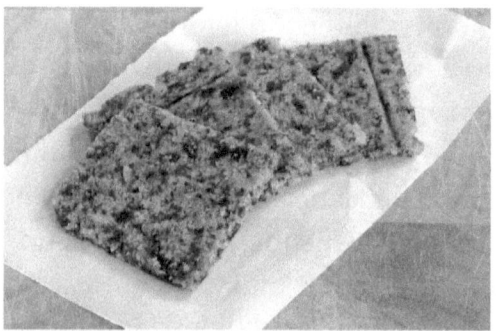

Easy-to-Make, Tangy Snacks to Keep You Healthy

Paleo Tortilla Chips – They are easy to make and ideal snacks to enjoy with homemade guacamole. This healthy, classic combo can be served to everyone in your family. These chips are made of almond flour. You can serve these healthy Paleo chips with other snacks on the bowl to have an unforgettable get-together next weekend. They are usually made with golden flax meal, almond flour, salt and egg whites.

Homemade Mango Salsa – It consists of fresh chopped mangos, cilantro, cucumber and scallion. This vivid Mexican salsa is the perfect combo of vitamins and proteins to fulfill your daily nutritional needs.

Paleo Chai Latte – It keeps you comfortable during the cold weather as it is made with Ayurvedic spices. The spices used in this drink are cardamom, cloves and cinnamon. It is an amazing on-the-go brunch. You can serve it as a healthy breakfast. It will give you great energy boost without caffeine.

Frozen Banana Bites – The specialty of these banana bites is that they are dipped with hot chocolate. This is a perfect choice to impress your partner on Valentine's Day. This chocolate dessert can save more time in the kitchen and lets you spend the same with your family. These choco-dipped banana slices are irresistible. The recipe of making this dessert is super simple and healthy.

5.4   It's Time for Dinner Party – Healthy and Tasty Gluten Free Dinner Ideas

As you know, people choose gluten-free diet because of several reasons. Most people, with a celiac condition are unable to absorb the gluten. Some people choose to experiment or implement gluten-free food in order to cleanse the body, refresh the immune system and stay healthy. Gluten-free food regime is also used and recommended in healing with various health conditions, for example in order to reduce inflammation and certain health problems.

Here are some healthy gluten-free dinner ideas and ingredients that you can use in gluten-free dinner.

Pasta Dishes and Casseroles

Since gluten-free meals avoid several grains, you might think that you don't have any option, but you would have a lot of choices and endless varieties. You can try making casseroles with rice if you are obsessed with it. Rice can be the best base for them because rice is gluten-free. You can buy gluten-free pasta from the health food stores and pick from the aisles of supermarkets. Gluten-free pastas are made with corn flour or rice. Several canned foods, such as creams, sauces, soups etc. have gluten. So, be wary with the ingredients you are adding in casseroles.

Gluten Free Sweet Potato Salad

Sweet Potato Salad with cinnamon raisin bread is the all-time staple for dinner party and barbeques. In this version, you have to use sweet potatoes for sweet, light recipe, which can be used either a hearty meal in the bowl or a side dish. You can serve this dish at room temperature or warm. It is versatile dish for hot meals on the balmy day or cool and soothing spring nights. Both you and your family will adore it. You can add extra taste with cinnamon raisin bread. To improve the sweetness you can add honey sauce on the potatoes and raisins. Add Sriracha sauce to add a bit of heat.

Make sure to avoid soy sauce because it contains gluten. However, gluten-free variant is also available in health food stores. You can enjoy delicious delight for dinner of potatoes mixed with gluten-free soy sauce.

Roasted Veggie Ragout & Shaved Parmesan

This vegetable ragout is a great option to savor the warming taste. It is the vegan's favorite option to feel fuller and satisfied. This soul food is easy to prepare and enjoy. It can be served with broiled polenta, hot pasta or steamed brown rice.

Parched Brown Rice Risotto

It is known as parched due to its rich texture. It is stirred for longer time on the stove. You can bake the brown rice with a great punch on flavor. It would be better if you have slivered, toasted almonds at hand. You can definitely have the disparity with soft baked rice with an added crunch. You can top it with nuts, cheese, or chopped parsley and serve in shallow bowls.

Gluten Free Pizza

If you are missing your favorite chili pizza just because you have no gluten-free option around, there is good news for you! You can make your own gluten-free pizza at home. It can have superior taste with perfect texture. It is not too thin and not too thick. The recipe of making it is pretty simple and ingredients are easily available.

Ingredients for Gluten-Free Staples

Beans

Several gluten-free beans are the perfect source of nutrients and vitamins, along with proteins. You can buy ready-to-make, canned black beans, fava beans, soy beans, red beans, navy beans and garbanzo beans, in dried form. You can add packaged flours made of such beans on certain recipes. Several specialty markets offer bean flour.

Gluten-Free Flour

It is important for those who are diagnosed with celiac disease. Rice flour, bean flour, corn flour and potato flour are the variants that replace traditional flour. You can pick the right type for your dinner recipes.

Tree Nuts

They don't have gluten and are rich in healthy fats and protein. They include almonds, peanuts, filberts, Brazil nuts, pecans and cashews. You can eat tree nuts roasted, raw or cooked with oils or butters, without mixing any ingredients that have gluten. If you have severe gluten intolerance, you should eat raw tree nuts.

Fresh Vegetables

They are naturally free from gluten. They have all the vital nutrients and vitamins required by your body for proper functioning. Avoid marinated veggies with gluten-free meals.

Rice

Some rice varieties are gluten-free, such as jasmine rice, basmati rice, black rice, japonica rice, brown rice, red rice, enriched rice calrose rice, and Arborio rice. Some rice varieties are used in Asian dishes and risotto dishes. You can happily eat these rice varieties. Avoid items made of farina, durum and wheat.

CHAPTER 6

Common Mistakes in Gluten-Free Diet You Should Avoid

Gluten is very harmful for those diagnosed with celiac disease. Some can severely weaken your body even more and most lead to reactions like illness and vomiting, diarrhea, unexpected weight loss. Gluten can affect small intestine and therefore practically all digestion system.

Eliminating gluten from the diet can control the disease and cope up with its symptoms and conditions. Many people tend to make some deadly mistakes when it comes to adopt gluten-free diet. In this chapter, we are going to discuss some of these mistakes and errors, so that you can be aware and instantly prepared to avoid them. Awareness means a lot, it can really safe you from lot of complications and trouble.

Having Blind Faith on Labels

Foods that are certified as "Gluten Free" and related labels, doesn't really mean that they are completely free of gluten. It's just like in example of as well popular "Fat Free" labeled meals – those (most of them out there on the market) are not actually fat free. Food industry corporations, large-scale food manufacturers, major regulatory loopholes and smart lawyers made this tricky situation probable and possible.

Many times this is exactly why most people with gluten allergy often ask themselves, "I am consuming gluten-free food for several months. Why I do not see anything improved. Why I still feel bad?"

According to existing FDA standards, manufacturers are allowed to add at least 20-PPM (Parts Per Million) gluten in their "Gluten Free" products. Even worse, certain foods that are labeled as "Gluten Free" are basically processed with sugar, rancid oils, and thickening agents. Now you may want to ask, "Why would these companies intentionally add such oils?" Oils like canola, corn, sunflower, safflower and soy have high amount of PUFAs (Polyunsaturated Fatty Acids), which go unstable in extraction process. These fatty acids prevent the healing process when you are trying to recover from allergies and gluten sensitivities.

On the other side, certain thickening agents like sorghum, guar gum, arrowroot, and rice starch can cause totally different complications. Anyone with gluten intolerance is losing the ability to absorb other foods properly. In such cases, thickening agents like starches are almost indigestible for the body. They decay in the gut and add pathogenic bacteria, which cause damage to the digestion system.

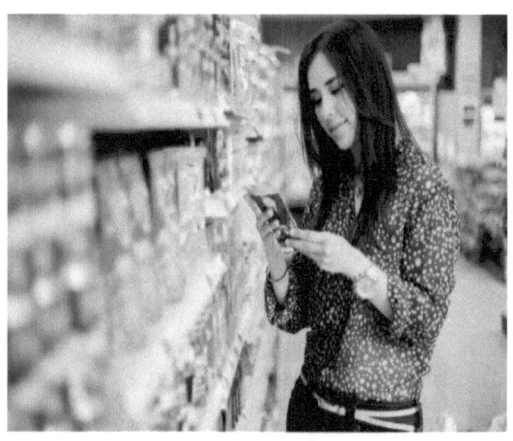

Assuming Foods Not Mentioning "Gluten" are Safe

Another common error we hope you are not trapped in. If you are not sure, please reconsider how you select foodstuff you are purchasing. For example, Gluten is added as stabilizing agent in ice cream and ketchups. If gluten is added during manufacturing process, gluten is often added on the food without mentioning it as an ingredient on the label. You might be shocked to know that your shampoo, tomato ketchup and even 100% Gluten-Free toast contains gluten. Here are the products and sources where gluten is found.

- **Cosmetics and Personal Care** – Soaps, shampoos, lipsticks, deodorants, all-natural sprays for hair, lotions, and even hand sanitizer have gluten as hydrolyzed wheat protein, wheat germ oil, hydrolyzed oat protein, oats, and textured plant protein.

- **Certain Supplements and Vitamins** – Around 25% of such products are cross contaminated with gluten-based ingredients.

- **Bulk Bins –** Raw walnuts and dried mangos are stored on the bin, which normally held oats, cereals and cornmeal and are probably not decontaminated in total and gluten safe manner.

- **Restaurants –** Even though restaurants show the menu, which contains gluten-free meals, they are not entirely gluten free and safe. It's most of the time not intentional off course but that isn't going to help you if you are not aware of it. For instance, the restaurant in your city or hotel you are visiting while you travel is serving contain gluten-free bread. However, when you take a "wide-angle look" then you can see, they are placing your gluten-free bread on the toaster where the other type of breads was getting toasted.

Giving up because committing to a Gluten-Free Diet is not easy

Eating in restaurants involves a lot of research. Restaurants that honestly provide

100% gluten-free are very rare. Gluten-free pizza is carried with same peel that is used to handle wheat one for another order.

Baking gluten-free on your own is like doing your own experiments and expecting the best. There are higher chances of running to mistakes.

But you should always keep in mind that all these problems are worth of trouble because gluten-free meals are very effective in recovery, if done in proper way.

Not Checking Labels in Grocery Shopping

This is already in a way covered; yet there is more to it. On gluten-free diet, some items that should really not be there are beer, pasta, processed meat, cereals, bread, crackers, condiments and ketchups. Gluten is found in several products and majority of people, even 'health food educated' consumers are not aware of it. For that reason, we are emphasizing the importance of this common error.

Simply make yourself enough eager and allow yourself to read labels on food packages, jars etc. properly and thoughtfully. You will be amazed to learn that even some toothpastes and lip balms contain gluten as binding agents. It off course depends on severity of your condition but regardless, even slight trace of Gluten can lead to severe reactions. So, it is better to avoid all the ingredients, all possibilities and just anything that may cause a reaction.

Thinking 'Gluten Free' and 'Wheat Free'

As we have been discussing in earlier chapters, gluten is not just found in wheat. There are many patients out there who report following gluten free diet, but in reality what they actually do is just replacing white bread and other foods with whole grain ones, which may have rye (that contain gluten) and spelt (belongs to wheat family). Naturally, all man, women and children that are not affected by gluten sensitivity and celiac disease conditions may feel great by having these in a diet – whole grains improve satiety and make one feels more energetic by allowing better and long lasting control of the insulin and blood sugar levels. They are for sure goodies but only for those not suffering from this any type of the gluten intolerance.

Dining Out Without Taking (Enough) Caution

Again, we all know that eating outside of home and safe environment can be risky. But for many individuals across US, Europe and rest of the world that are living with the gluten intolerance, dealing properly with this is just *very, very important.*

Normally, most of the menus are made of dishes, which do contain gluten. If the restaurant is not offering Gluten Free menu, it is better to ask the chef or the personal for possibility of gluten-free dishes. You off course have limited choices and if you are already battling this health condition and you are dinning out, you know how complex this may be.

Restaurant owners (as well as chefs, waiters and waitresses) are not to blame for that. There are just too many implications to cover. Flour is used to thicken the sauces and some of the dressings. Make sure you do not order some of those. Normally, one can adjust to this regiment in 2-3 weeks of practice but 'success rate' and ease really depends on a place you are visiting.

'Choice of the restaurant, dinner or hotel is therefore more important that what you can order once you are there'.

Common sense steps of avoiding cross-contamination (sharing bread knife, avoiding left crumbs of bread in butter, etc.) are off course important.

Misunderstanding Gluten Free with Weight Loss

Now this may not be relevant to you but you would be amazed how many people this one affects. News and media are sometimes serving the information about a celebrity, (or you may heard about a coworker or a friend) who suddenly lose significant amount of weight by giving up gluten.

Actually, this is not how they (or anyone else) got to a success in a weight loss. One cannot think about the Gluten free diet as a weight loss diet – simply do not consider it as one and the same because they are not. On top of everything else, healthy weight loss occurs by avoiding foods that contain high amount of refined carbs like pasta, bagels, pretzels, crackers, and baked goods. In fact, adopting gluten free diet may also increase the weight.

Excess to 'Gluten-Free' Junk Food

This is very connected to the previous point. Gluten free meals have been enjoying increasing popularity in last couple of years. Hence, dozens of gluten-free variants are available in the markets nowadays, such as gluten-free variants of carb-laden pasta, bagels, pretzels, crackers and baked items. Now, did you notice for example that some of the popular gluten-free cookies have about 60 calories per each 1 piece? It is surprisingly more than a normal sandwich cookie, right?

All in all, just going gluten-free doesn't assure the loss of inches and pounds.

Verdict

People diagnosed with celiac disease, are recommended to live 100% gluten-free. Only some people in this category can eat gluten without suffering from the negative side effects.

For most of us, allowing Gluten to creep in to our lunches, dinners and other meals is risky because even a small trace of gluten can cause very adverse effects and worsening the illness. Gluten-free diets may cause mineral and vitamin deficits as grains have certain nutrients like folate, iron, fiber and calcium.

If done in right way Gluten-free life can be interesting and not too restrictive, austere, or isolating. One has to learn and develop a habit of looking for foods that are naturally gluten-free. Also, you have to be playful and keep experimenting alternative recipes until you find the best one that suits you and your family, guests, clients or who ever is going to enjoy the food you are preparing.

CHAPTER 7

Adopting a Gluten-Free Lifestyle Effortlessly

A lot of gluten-free products are there in the market today. Some people conclude that avoiding gluten is the best and healthy choice for their lifestyle. Some people choose gluten-free lifestyle yet doctors recommend gluten-free diet only to those diagnosed with celiac disease. A lot of people who adopted gluten free diet claim that they have improved their health and feel better.

People tend to believe that they have celiac disease just because they have gastrointestinal problems. Reliable doctor and medical specialists will never recommend gluten-free diet to a patient until undergoing in depth and proper diagnosis.

It is important - you shouldn't start consuming 100% gluten-free food until you actually are clear about your condition. Now, once you are diagnosed and sure you are having Gluten intolerance or allergy, there are things that will immensely help you. For example, just because you've seen gluten-free foods in the aisles of health food stores, it doesn't really mean they are completely safe. It is unfortunate and sort of irrational yet reality shows us that some gluten-free products have high amount of fat and sugar, which are not at all helpful for those with celiac disease.

Cross contamination is another important issue for people who want to adopt gluten-free diet. Here is one of the classical examples of a cross-contamination:

Suppose a housewife is making sandwiches for her two children - one has celiac disease and another one is healthy.

When it comes to spread jam, she uses same knife on both gluten-free and gluten-containing bread. In that way, gluten particles are easily transferred into the gluten-free bread. Similarly, as we already have listed in previous chapters, those cocking and serving the food in the hotels and restaurants have to know and assure gluten free environment that is safe of cross contamination as well. It is important for entire personal (not only the chefs) to arrange for and use separate utensils, pots, working areas. Not many are aware about this and so are not arranging enough steps in this direction. Others however (there are great examples you will meet) are really strict and expertly cook and prepare the foods in separate kitchens meant for preparation of the gluten-free meals.

The Gluten free diet and lifestyle is important for dealing with serious and real health problems faced by many man and women affected by gluten intolerance, gluten allergy and celiac disease.

According to the recent statistics, around 18 million US residents are suffering from gluten intolerance, gluten allergy or celiac disease (and tendency of increasing seem to be quite strong). Here are few main 'dos and don'ts' that are maybe practical before getting started with gluten-free diet.

Dos
- Check Food Labels
- Learn everything about gluten
- Ensure buying "Gluten-Free" certified products
- Eat a lot of unprocessed, fresh foods
- Study the Inner Healing approach
- Be consistent in Outer and Inner approach

Don'ts
- Don't avoid informing your family and friends about your dietary problems
- Don't eat out and order processed meals

- Don't cross contaminate
- Avoid alcohol beverages

Do's

Study Everything about Gluten Intolerance

You have to know your enemy. For winning the war, it is not enough just to know 'something' about the enemy, starting from the basics such as these:

Gluten is a specific type of protein found in rye, wheat and barley. If you are sensitive to Gluten, you might suffer some symptoms like bloating, constipation, reduced digestion and diarrhea. It can cause severe weight loss and malnutrition. Person needs proper diagnosis in order to determine if you have celiac disease or not. Gluten intolerance or sensitivities are related to several digestive issues and bloating, headaches or migraines, brain fog, joint pains, eczema and chronic tiredness, and skin irritations.

On contrary to modern medicine claims, one can significantly improve the health condition and even heal entirely by taking to complete approach to Gluten free lifestyle.

Check Food Labels

Is it easy finding out which foods have gluten and which doesn't? Sometimes yes, very often not! While pasta, wheat bread, and flour are obvious and known to contain gluten, there are some foods don't seem to contain gluten, but they actually do.

Some of these processed foods, average person would never

place in a gluten-containing category: soy sauce, cooking spray, mustard, salad dressing and flavored yogurt are just few examples. According to FDA, food makers have to mention 8 most popular ingredients on labels, which are related to food allergies like eggs, milk, fish, nuts, peanuts, soy, shellfish and wheat and yet many do not follow this rule or they do by using very tiny size of the text on the boxes and labels, so have your reading glasses ready.

Another thing: technically, gluten is not an allergic ingredient. Hence, manufacturers often don't list it. So, when shopping, it is much better that you should check the label for the ingredients that contain gluten, such as soy, wheat and even gelatin, etc.

Eat Proper Amount of Unprocessed, Fresh Foods

As a rule of thumb, if you want healthy eating and are on gluten-free diet, you should pick products from the 'outer aisles'. This is basically because almost all the vegetables and fruits in such areas are not processed and have fewer chances to contain gluten. However, some processed foods like most gluten-free potato chips are safe to eat.

Search for Products Certified as "Gluten Free"

According to the new FDA regulations as of August 2014, all the products with labels "Without Gluten", "Gluten Free", "No Gluten" or "Free of Gluten" may contains at least 20 PPM Gluten. So, you should search for gluten-free products certified by any third-party organization proving that company performs correct processes to avoid any gluten contamination and to keep the gluten levels below 20 PPM.

The companies have to opt for gluten-free compliance standard to earn the certification. They also have to undergo on-site inspections of handling and manufacturing process along with product testing every year. Hence, consumers are rest assured with food that has been processed through gluten-free supply chain and has below 20 PPM of gluten.

Study the Inner Healing Approach

If you want to enjoy a full and happy life, you shouldn't (like most of people with Gluten intolerance and celiac) rely only on the outer approach.

Yes, you need to address the diet in very strict and accurate way. And yes, it is very important and it is not totally easy thing to do. In the same time however, that is NOT going to heal you. You have to address the causes of your condition and with good methods (like the one we are underline(presenting in this book) you will for sure get what others don't – full and happy Gluten free life style.

Be consistent

In order to make sure you are not risking your health and not wasting your time you just have to develop a habit of being consistent. You should not allow being 'seasonal'. Stick to the diet and health-boosting practices you chose to follow. Don't give up on those.

Don'ts

Don't Forget Informing Family and Friends about Your Problem

For a person with gluten sensitivity or intolerance, it can be very difficult if other family members don't have the same problem. That doesn't mean you should keep them unaware about your condition and your dietary needs.

Whether you are eating at your friend's house, ensure that your family or friends know what to serve you and what is off-limit for your diet. Life is much easier in that way.

Don't Cross-Contaminate

Whether you are sharing kitchen with the person who don't have issue with gluten or you have just adopted gluten-free life, you must think about preventing cross-contamination with dishes, food and utensils. It is better to keep separate dishes and silverware for preparing gluten-free food. Also clean the spaces like stoves, counters and fridge shelves completely.

Don't Try to Eat Unprepared in Restaurants

As you know, some restaurants provide quite opulent choice of gluten free dishes and some don't. When it comes to ordering your favorite goodies, be sure you are aware and attentive. You can check online menu out, before heading to your favorite restaurant.

Don't hesitate to ask the server about certain dishes and their ingredients.

Don't Drink Alcoholic Beverages

If you are on a gluten-free diet, make sure to avoid ale, beer and stout. Also try to avoid light rum, vodka and wine, unless they are certified gluten free.

Verdict

To sum up, gluten free diet is medically recommended to those people who have celiac disease or gluten allergy. If you have such problems, you should be properly informed about gluten and facts about it. Even though you are adopting gluten-free diet just as a choice, you still should consider these tips and the above dos and don'ts to ensure doing it in right way. Keep in mind that gluten-free diet is especially recommended for those who have gluten sensitivity or have celiac disease.

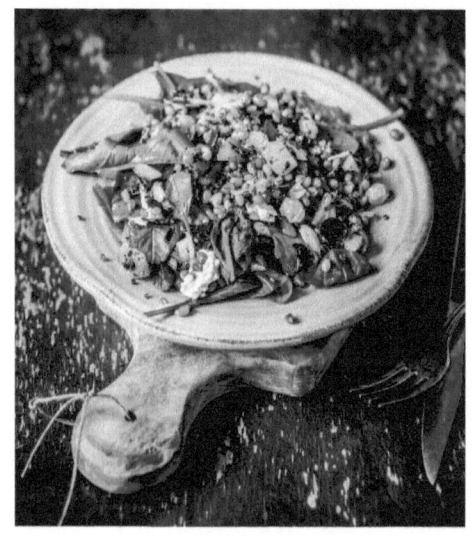

CHAPTER 8

Other Tips & Suggestions

Getting diagnosed with celiac disease or gluten allergy can be frustrating and overwhelming experience. Dietitians and doctors recommend a long list of foods to eat and avoid. But they don't discuss the strategies of how to live painlessly. In this chapter, I am going to discuss surprising and easiest ways to live normal lifestyle without gluten.

8.1 How Do I Know If Certain Food is Gluten-Free?

As we know, Gluten is a type of protein basically associated with wheat and found in some grains. Before getting in to this health condition, people do not even think about the gluten, sensitivity to it or gluten allergy. You may as well remember yourself, wandering about Gluten Free label etc. Now, all related to Gluten free lifestyle probably is (or it should be) extra important to you. That is natural.

We are surrounded by foods containing gluten and wheat. Let us list steps you should be willing to follow in order to determent whether or not the food is gluten-free.

Know the type of products or grains that contain gluten. Gluten is mainly found in rye, wheat, buckwheat, barley, bulgur, bran, millet, wheat germ and etc. Gluten can also be found in foods fermented or processed with gluten-based products like wheat flour. Hence, the ideal way is that you should know the ingredients that have gluten.

Check the Labels Entirely

Ensure that you buy gluten-free products by checking out the labels, which have ingredients. Flours made with coconut, corn and rice are gluten-free alternatives to wheat flour.

Know About the Labels

See the packaging. With the popularity and demand of gluten-free products, the manufacturers started adding the phrases like "No Added Gluten" or "Gluten Free". Typically it will be seen on the packaging. The companies have to follow FDA regulations to offer gluten-free products.

Buy products only from a reliable source. Some companies are intended and focused on offering only gluten-free products and you can also buy them online. Several health food stores have gluten-free product ranges.

Home Food

Make your own meals more often. You can make the gluten-free food on your own which is best way to ensure gluten-free diet regiment. You can find a lot of gluten free recipes all around and undoubtedly you will be assured with ingredients when you are the one who mixes, cooks or bakes them.

8.2 Eating Gluten Free at Restaurants

For some people, going gluten-free is just a healthy choice. But for man and women with celiac disease or gluten insensitivity, it's a need. Hence, it is important to develop skills of avoiding foods that contain gluten. Though in the beginning, it may feel almost impossible to live without eating gluten-based foods, one can adjust to living without gluten in relatively short time. For most it isn't quite easy road but it gets easier as you invest effort.

When it comes to dining out, self-control is crucial element and that is at times fairly difficult. But with these tips and ideas may help you:

- Ask the waiter or waitress for a gluten-free menu. People have become more aware about celiac disease and gluten intolerance over the last few years. For that reason, more restaurants and food chains are offering gluten-free food options and meals.

- Use your browsing skills on computer or mobile phone and see if restaurant you are planning to visit is offering gluten-free meals or not. Visit to regular menu page is normally good way to start – you may find a notation such as "Gluten-Free Meals Available" or a separate section where those options are listed.

- Increase the attention of the personal by informing the waiter about your gluten-allergy or celiac disease. After getting aware about your health condition, they will be extra-caring towards you and your nutritional needs.

- Tell the waiter not to add bread on your plate. Eating bread seems tempting and avoiding it while having the fresh slices bellow your nose, sometimes can be real torture. Even worse, some patients actually report having a reaction with just smell of fresh gluten containing bread.

- Warn the restaurant personal not to add croutons or dressing on salad. If you are salad enthusiasts you may think about having your favorite bottle of salad dressing, naturally free of gluten. Carry it in your handbag or purse.

- Order the steamed rice. Along with being delicious, rice is the great alternative to wheat and it is great fit to different recipes. Typically, it is good to know about variety of meals and dished that are rice based or can be combined with a rice. Also, rice bread and rice flour is great replacement for wheat flour and wheat bread.

- Some of you may not really enjoy this idea and yet, I know many people that find this one really great and helpful in practice, especially if you like the place and you plan to visit again. Tip your waiter higher than it is a customary or normal, i.e. at least 30% of the bill. Though it is higher than normal tip, it is best deal to have good waiter or waitress who can take your dietary needs seriously.

Gluten-Free Desserts

Finding suitable desert options sometimes can be really difficult. Naturally, ice cream (most of it) is gluten-free. The processing part in some brands is different and gluten is added in the late phases. Be aware of that as well. Now, you will find more but let us share with you just several brands that still offer finger-licking gluten-free desserts.

TCBY

The Country's Best Yogurt (TCBY) lists some of the best products made without gluten. They offer mostly gluten-free ice creams. The only problem is cross-contamination in ice cream parlors. Make sure the server serves you after washing off the ice-cream scoop. This way, you can eliminate the risk of accidentally eating traces of gluten.

Baskin-Robbins

It is yet another brand that mentions all the allergen details on all of its ice-cream containers. The company maintains solid level of transparency by listing all ice creams that don't have wheat. But they don't point out rye, barley or oats on their products. So, one can determine such ingredients on case-by-case basis. As a general rule of thumb, you can eat most of the ice creams of that brand. They don't offer any product on sandwich or cone as they have gluten.

Skinny Cow

If you are a celiac and want to monitor your weight and maintain healthy living, it is good to enjoy ice creams of Skinny Cow. See the list of their products and choose the one you love.

Trader Joe's

They provide a huge range of frozen desserts and they have "Gluten-Free Ingredients List". Their menu has something for every celiac.

8.3 Add These Gluten-Free Foods in Your Diet

For us who are facing the complexities of celiac disease, it is really very important to make strong decision and stick to a decision not to eat anything that contains gluten. As you probably know from your own experience, at first it may seem overwhelming and too demanding. Once you learn what is important and what not, once you get accustomed with reading labels and choosing food items that are gluten-free, you can start enjoying a healthy and well-balanced diet, which is loaded with rich taste.

Rice

Some of the rice varieties, come in the market, are gluten-free. You may not want to eat some varieties because of the fear of cross contamination. Some varieties like japonica, jasmine, basmati, calrose, Arborio, black rise, brown rise etc. are used to make risotto dishes and some glutinous varieties are covered in gluten-free recipes. But you should avoid other items like bulgur that are made of couscous, wheat, farina and durum.

Gluten-Free Flour

For anyone with gluten sensitivity and celiac disease, gluten-free flour is important ingredient. Living without flour, for most of us is just hard. Fortunately there are options and tasty substitutes. Types of gluten-free flours, such as rice flour, bean flour, potato flour, soy flour, and corn flour should become part of your shopping list. You can experiment with various recipes and choose the perfect kind of flour for your cooking and dietary needs.

Fresh Veggies

Naturally, this comes with no surprise. Fresh veggies are grown gluten-free and they have all the vital nutrients and vitamins needed for proper functioning of our bodies. However, you should avoid marinated vegetables and similar varieties of dishes unless you ensure that they are processed with gluten-free elements.

Tree Nuts

Tree nuts have 'best of both worlds' – they are rich in healthy fats and protein and they don't have gluten. You can have almonds, peanuts, filberts, Brazil nuts, and pecans. You can eat them roasted, raw or made with oils or butters until they are not blended with elements that have gluten. You should choose raw nuts labeled as gluten-free if you have severe sensitivity with gluten.

Beans

Several beans are rich source of protein and are free of gluten. They also have other vital nutrients and vitamins. You can have red beans, Fava beans, black beans, soybeans, red beans and navy beans. They are quite easy to prepare can be used in many delicious recipes.

8.4 Gluten-Free Grains

For anyone with gluten allergy and sensitivity, gluten-free grains are as well very important. Some information's sources will tell you that oats re the best. Yes, oats are normally gluten-free but they are widely processed with gluten-based ingredients. Anyhow, here are some of the gluten-free grains that can fulfill all your dietary needs.

Millet

Funny thing you may be aware of, in the US, they are basically used as birdseed. But in other countries like China, South America, Africa and India, it is considered as staple grain. Millet has high amount of minerals like phosphorus, iron and calcium. It comes from a grass whose grains are red, yellow, white or grey. It also has higher protein and lysine than rice, corn and oats. It has a delicate taste and it can be coupled with other grains and toasted to improve versatility.

Buckwheat

You may use buckwheat cracked, whole or as flour. Its seed is triangular shaped. Irrespective of its name, it has no relation with wheat, but it is in fact related to rhubarb. Regardless, you should read the labels carefully because it may be mixed with wheat products. Buckwheat is probably the best alternative for pasta if it is in its white, whole form. It gets its burnt, nutty flavor as roasted, kasha buckwheat. Buckwheat has all the vital amino acids and it in deed great choice.

Montina

Well, many of you did not taste or have any experience with this one, right? Montina is made with Indian rice grass and can be combined with or milled in the flours to form a baking mix. It is sort of aromatic 'woodsy' in taste and it is green in color. Montina is another great gluten-free option, rich in fiber and protein.

Quinoa

The South America's staple grain, quinoa is totally a protein food that is normally cooked fluffy and it is like Swiss chard. The grains may be black, purple, red or light hued. The outer part carries the bitter saponins that should be cleaned off. For some hot dishes, you can use it whole, also as an alternative of other grains, and as flour.

8.5. 7-Day Gluten-Free Meal Plan

It is easy to get frustrated and overwhelmed in order to plan meals for those who have gluten sensitivity. Meal planning can be more challenging for busy modern world women, especially when it comes to personalizing meal plans for gluten-free needs. In reality, pre-planned meal plan can make your life a lot easier and cooking much happier experience.

Despite this guide isn't a cookbook or a diet plan, we think that it may inspire you to get more ideas on your own. Once you start getting along with more experience and your own ideas start flowing, you will be no longer frustrated or confused.

For the beginning, try out this 7-day meal plan.

Day – 1 (Sunday)

Breakfast – Instant Gluten-free Taco and Honeydew melon (1 cup)

Lunch – Gluten-free Pizza, Skim milk (1 cup)
Dinner – Traditional Vegetable Soup, Rice Pilaf, Zucchini with Squash
For Snacking – Chewable Gluten-Free Granola Bars (Dairy Free, Egg Free and Vegan), Banana-Blackberry Ice Cream, and fresh baby carrots

Day -2 (Monday)

Breakfast – Apple Raisin and Pumpkin Oatmeal, 1 cup skim milk
Lunch – Gluten free buckwheat bread, chopped juicy cauliflower salad, strawberries (1 cup)
Dinner – Szechuan Peanut Noodles served with broccoli , Sweet potato (baked), cooked quinoa (1/2 CUP)
Snacking – Quinoa Almond Bars and 1 ½ cup air popped popcorn

Day – 3 (Tuesday)

Breakfast – GF Granola with Mulberries and Walnuts, Green Creamy Smoothie with a few Hints of Mint
Lunch – Spicy Tropical Salsa and Baked Tilapia, 1 cup skim milk
Dinner – Carrot and Rutabaga Puree, Salad, cooked brown rice (1/2 cup), low-fat vanilla yogurt
Snacks/Dessert – Sugar-free and Gluten-free Chocolaty Vanilla cupcakes

Day – 4 (Wednesday)

Breakfast – Sweet Potato Pancakes, 1 cup skim milk, grapefruit and fortified breakfast cereal (Gluten-Free)
Lunch – Risotto, tortilla and papaya
Dinner – Cilantro Crema and Avocado Tacos, 1 small apple, low-fat cheddar cheese (1 Oz)
Snacking/Dessert – Cookie Bars with Choco chips, Strawberry Cheesecake (dairy free and gluten free)
Day – 5 (Thursday)

Breakfast – Potato Parsley Pancakes
Lunch – Avocado Tacos
Dinner – Stuffed Green Peppers
Snacking/Dessert – Lemon Frozen
Yogurt, Gluten-Free and Dairy Free
Pumpkin Spice Muffins

Day – 6 (Friday)

Breakfast – Blueberry Pancakes (Gluten
Free), Custom Fruit Salad
Lunch – Grass-fed Burger
Dinner – Crust-less Vegetable Quiche
Snacking/Dessert – Delicious dense
brownies (dairy/casein free and gluten
free), baked apple chips

Day – 7 (Saturday)

Breakfast – Banana Pomegranate Ginger
Blast
Lunch – Black bean burritos
Dinner – Zucchini Gratin and Eggplant

Snacking/Dessert – Pumpkin Cheesecake

DISCLAIMER

Though all the steps have been taken to provide in-depth, effective and accurate information in the book "Happy & Gluten Free -Lifestyle Guide", neither the publisher nor the author is responsible for inaccuracies, errors, or omissions. Any sights of organization or people are unintentional.

This guide is published with an intention to help people with celiac disease kick-start their gluten-free diet and to learn about foods that are naturally gluten-free. However, readers are requested to ask the nutrition expert, dietitian or physician first before starting any diet. You may consider this guide as a complement step after seeing professional help. People who start their diet without any expert help may experience difficulty, frustration, confusion, and, even worse, depression.

Neither the author nor the publisher takes responsibility for any change in the information after publication from research.

The book should not be taken as a substitute to doctor's recommendation and the source of medical information. The book is designed to give authoritative and accurate information with regards to the subject matter herein. Those who purchase this book acknowledge that the publisher is not intended to offering any medical advice. For any kind of medical help, the reader is strongly recommended to seek professional help before following any step.

Published in United States of America

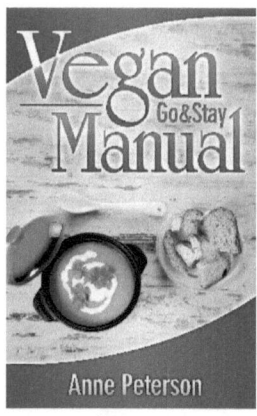

QUICK GUIDE to VEGAN DIET & LIFESTYLE - PRACTICAL MANUAL THAT WILL ASSIST YOUR 'GOING & STAYING VEGAN

Shop on Amazon

(You DON'T necessarily need a Kindle reader device in order use this book. It's available for immediate reading with your Amazon virtual cloud reader).

Author who surprised readership with Golfing guide for the beginners 'Lifesaving' ABC Golf Instruction is coming with even bigger surprise. Switching to Vegan diet almost three decades ago, Mrs. Peterson grow more and more passionate about Vegan lifestyle, promoting it and assisting others in various matters connected to Vegan diet and lifestyle. Anne has managed to channel three decades of experience in this short, practical and easy to use form. This manual is filled with great looking photographs that add to smooth mood of this manual.

WARNING: THIS is NOT a cookbook - if you are looking for a collection of recipes and nothing else, you probably do not want this book. HOWEVER - VEGAN (Go & Stay) Manual will definitely enthuse your (Vegan cooking) creativity and ideas plus it will do for you so much more. Offering 'down to earth' guidelines, practical information and advice focused on health and well-being, Anne Peterson is avoiding all fluff, philosophical approaches and theories (that we normally find in most of the Vegan books not based on recipes). No one has to be worried about the title - this work in fact is a Manual. VEGAN (Go & Stay) Manual is not going to help only those man ans women who consider switching to Veganism but even to those that are already familiar with theory and practice of Vegan way of living.

In essence, what you see in front of you is quite unique, short yet very useful peace of information.

Make practical use of well-known wisdom lines such as 'KNOWLEDGE is the POWER'. HEALTHY VEGAN = HAPPY VEGAN – link to book

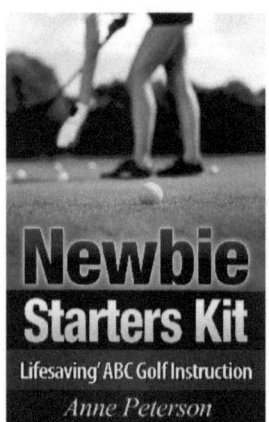

SIMPLE and DETAILED BEGGINERS GUIDE TO THE WORLD OF GOLF That will save YOUR TIME & MONEY

Shop on Amazon

Anyone new (or not too experienced) to a game of Golf will definitely benefit from this guide immensely. You can start reading this book on Kindle device or computer right away.

Unlike most Golf books we see around today, this guide is not presenting any sort of advanced knowledge, 'cool strategies, tactics and secrets'. Other books force a reader to turn in to 'more that he / she desires to be' – simple Golf lover and player for fun and enjoyment. Nothing like that you will find here. WHY? Well, nothing that is of sound quality, nothing really great or powerful in this world exists that without very firm and solid ground principles and basic knowledge. This really is a Newbie Starter Kit – simple yet fundamental for (any) Golfer.

I think you will agree with explanation how this book can boost up your Golfing carrier + safe you solid amounts of time and money. Here is just a thought: most people (not only newbies) fall pray to "ego trip" mind trick, mostly due to felling a social pressure. They start to artificially rush up the things in order to create illusion of "fast advancement" and in that way, many man and women miss to understand important aspects and gain basic understandings important for anyone who plays Golf. No amount of expensive special clothing and Golf gear can make you play better and no variety of cool tricks you learn from a book will help you either without having firm and solid BASIC UNDESRTANDING. So, I am not saying there is anything wrong with expensive gear and Golf clothes – I LOVE enjoying in those, as well. Out on the course, peace of mind is giving you more than all those things. In any case, If you consider yourself a beginner, nothing will help you more that simple and clear explanation of (practically) everything you need to know about and start your Golfing adventure.

SAFE YOUR TIME AND MONEY, KICKSTART YOU'RE GOLFING EXPERIENCE RIGHT NOW!

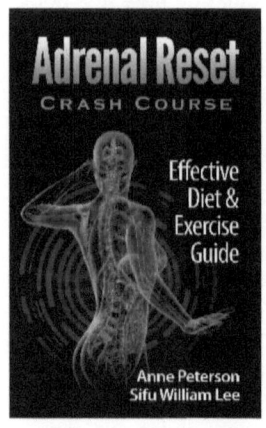

This Unique Approach to ADRENAL RESET DIET is SIMPLE and EFFECTIVE Solution to ADRENAL Fatigue & Poor Results in Fat Loss and Weight Management. Combined with Ancient Chinese Qigong (Free Video Included), it WILL Offer You Immediate Results & HELP you from Inside Out!

Sifu Lee's bestselling Amazon titles are helping and healing thousands of people – this book will do the same. Anne Peterson has the biggest qualification – started as mother of two children with developed gluten intolerance, she grew in to passionate protagonist of healthy diet and lifestyle. This guide is NOT for those searching for theories or medical statistics. It is loaded with practical and effective solutions, information and tips. Also, this is a COMBINED EFFORT: Having two children with gluten intolerance had forced Anne Peterson and her family to many tribulations, experimenting and searching for best ways to live on a gluten free diet.

That developed Anne to a level of expert in the field of nutrition, healthy diet and lifestyle. As a passionate protagonist of effective solutions, she had great advantage compared to someone without that deep knowledge and yet, new horizon's opened once she came in contact with Sifu William Lee.
HEALING from INSIDE OUT: Practices of Traditional Chinese Medicine (TCM) are by most people considered complicated for learning and applying. But, if you look any of the books written by Sifu Lee you will see different truth. Most of people who suffer from Adrenal fatigue do not even dream about possibility of being helped with anything but changes in diet. In this book, Sifu explains the basic facts and helps you to learn Qiqong meridian stretching routine trough a simple Video presentation. Regardless of who you are, if you are suffering from Adrenal fatigue (or you suspect you may be), you really need this guide. Anyone with open mind will benefit immensely from the tips, information, guidelines and practices presented within this great book.

Check NOW this EFFECTIVE Guide for FAST & SIMPLE Solution for ADRENAL FATIGUE!

Sifu William Lee

Amazon author Page

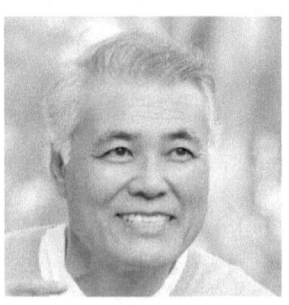

From early childhood on, I worked hard just to get food and water - times were extremely hard in Zhengzhou, China. When I was 5 years old, my mother had to leave my three sisters and me in order to survive. Though it seems like a terrible beginning, we all lived through it and gained great life experience. The will of providence brought me to work as a servant in the house of the great master, Sifu Qian Bo-Wan. His Kung Fu school became my home and shelter. At the age of 8, my passion for martial arts was recognized and I began learning personally from the great Bo-Wan.

I was trained in various methods: Wing Chun, Shao Lin Guan, Tai Chi Guan, Xing Xi Guam. I studied Chi Kung with my master and Buddhist monks. Just before my Sifu left this world, he told me: "Xi (his name for me), you have to go and spread this knowledge. You can do much more then I ever could, you will see." I felt humbled and obligated to carry out his wishes.

After finishing my studies of traditional Chinese medicine with Dr. Le Cai, I moved to the Western world. I have to admit, I never understood what my Sifu meant by 'you can do much more'. He did not say 'better', but more. I spent the last 30 years in teaching martial arts, Chi Kung, and related disciplines, but just recently I understood why he used the term 'much more'.

It was not because of anything in me. It is because of the Internet and modern technology that I really am able to fully fulfill his instructions. I am more than grateful to all my students and readers who help me, and continue reading and using my books. Thank you from the bottom of my heart, and God bless you.